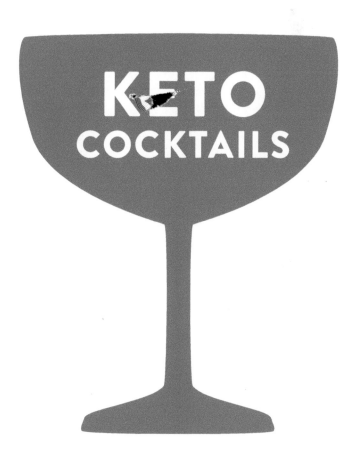

KETO
COCKTAILS

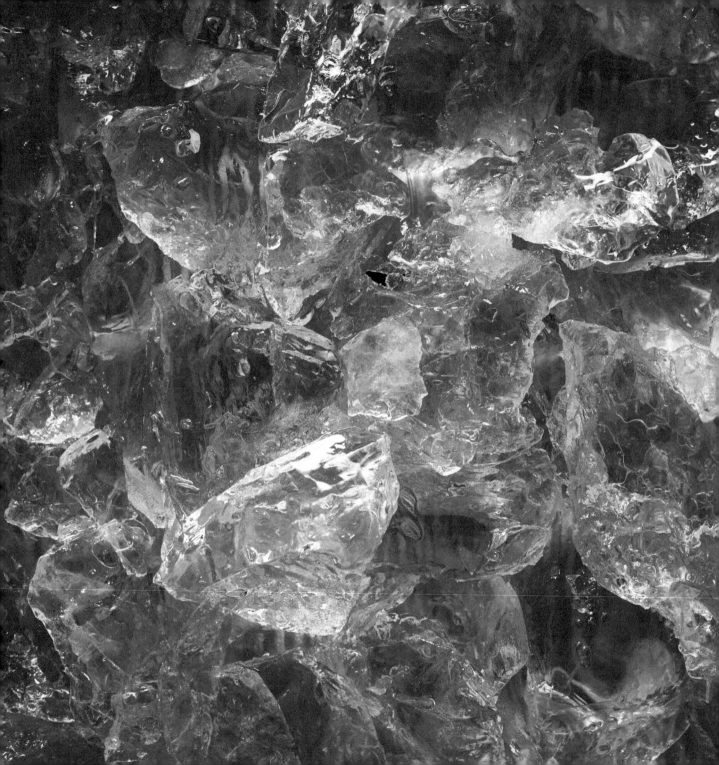

# KETO
## COCKTAILS
### 75 LOW-CARB LIBATIONS

TASHA METCALF

Photography by Iain Bagwell

ROCKRIDGE
PRESS

For general information on our other products and services or to obtain technical support, please contact our Customer Care Department within the United States at (866) 744-2665, or outside the United States at (510) 253-0500.

Rockridge Press publishes its books in a variety of electronic and print formats. Some content that appears in print may not be available in electronic books, and vice versa.

Interior and Cover Designer: Patricia Fabricant
Art Producer: Meg Baggott
Editor: Anna Pulley
Production Manager: Holly Haydash
Production Editor: Melissa Edeburn
Photography © 2020 Iain Bagwell. Food styling by Loren Wood.

ISBN: Print 978-1-64739-734-0 | eBook 978-1-64739-436-3
R0

For my grandparents, William and Beverly Steffen, who let me run wild at the Chieftain and play bartender with the soda gun and fountain dispensers growing up.

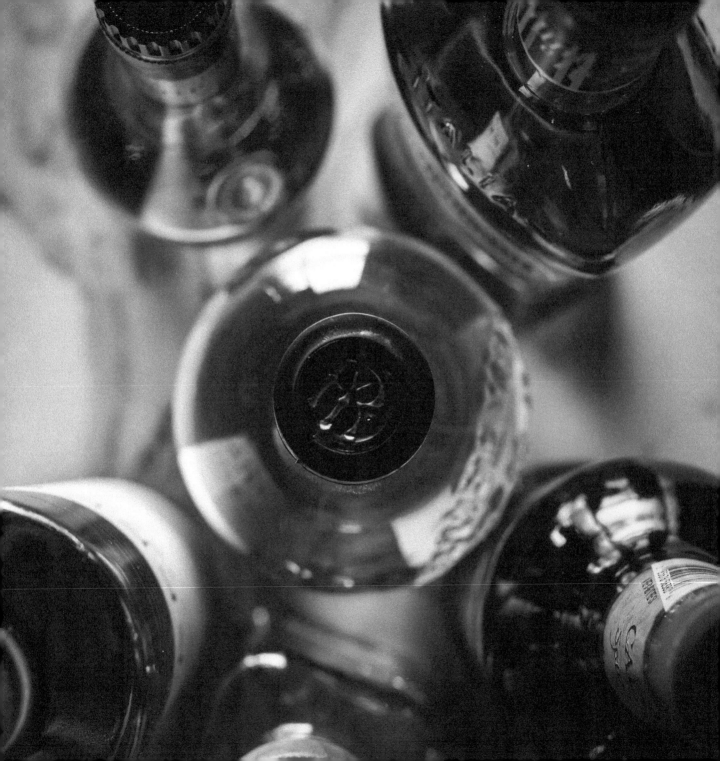

# CONTENTS

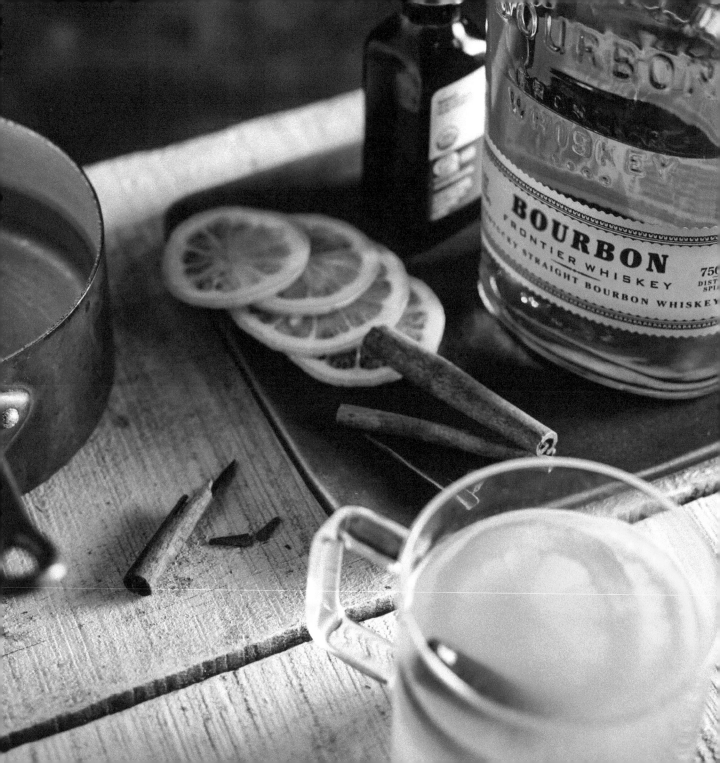

# INTRODUCTION

I grew up in a bar. Long before I learned how to mix drinks, barhop, or handle my liquor, I hung out on a barstool watching Saturday morning cartoons while my family buzzed around at work. It was there, at the family restaurant and bar, that I learned to cook and master the fine art of washing dishes. Though I wasn't able to serve alcohol, I spent my fair share of time behind the bar and could make a mean Shirley Temple—ginger ale and a splash of grenadine, with a cherry on top. My first official cocktail. Naturally, I moved on to more advanced (and boozy) drinks with age. Though I'm not a professional mixologist, I feel particularly well equipped to help navigate the confusing land of keto cocktails.

I've eaten low carb for years, even before "ketosis" became a household buzzword. I own and operate a private nutrition business that specializes in keto and low-carb dietary patterns, and I develop recipes and meal plans at Ketogasm.com. I've written two books about the keto diet and I studied nutrition in grad school. You, my friend, are in good hands.

I didn't always know what I was doing, though. Far from it. There were limited resources available when I was learning the ropes. When I tried hunting down suitable recipes for my favorite drinks, desserts, and comfort foods, they didn't exist. Popular opinion at the time was unanimously restrictive: "You can't have that anymore." As more of an "everything in moderation" kind of gal, I started developing my own keto-friendly versions of what everyone preached was off-limits. Eventually, I started sharing them. Turns out, there's a way to make just about everything keto, including cocktails.

This book is one I wish I had had years ago: a guide to mixing simple, delicious, keto-friendly cocktails. It covers the fundamentals of mixing low-carb drinks and presents keto versions of classic cocktails as well as innovative concoctions. It even includes tasty happy hour food and sometimes-spiked desserts. Whether you're a novice or seasoned mixologist, you'll find in this book all the tools you need to become an expert home bartender. I hope you have just as much fun reading this book as you do enjoying the recipes!

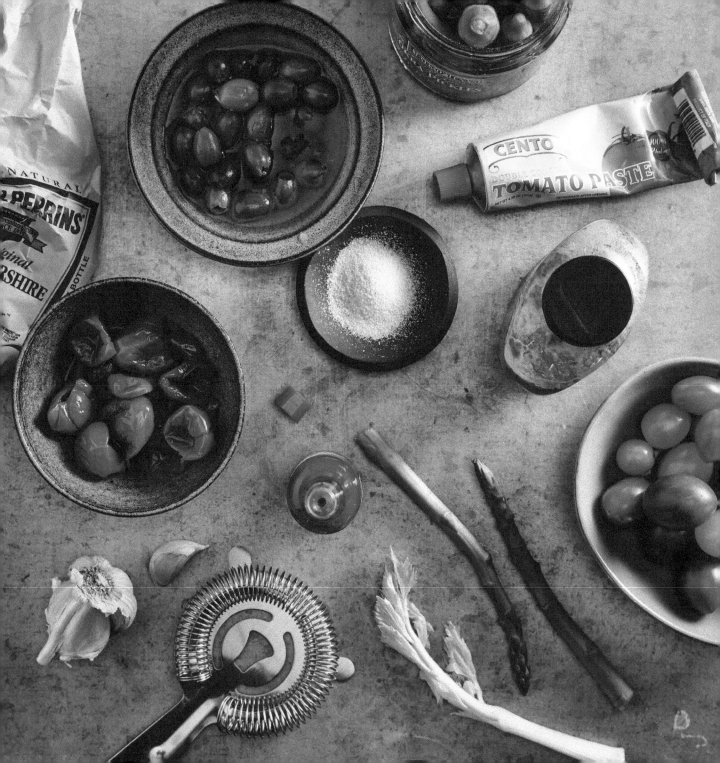

# = 1 =
# BOOZY BASICS: A KETO ALCOHOL PRIMER

Alcohol on keto? You better believe it, baby. To kick things off, we're brushing up on keto basics to set you up for success. Though it may be tempting to flip straight to the recipes, this chapter is overflowing with tips you won't want to miss. Here you'll find a quick refresher on keto and learn how alcohol affects the body in ketosis. In addition, you'll score time-tested hangover hacks (you'll thank me later) and a handy cheat sheet to help you cruise carb counts of different drinks, so you know when to turn up and when to run for the hills. Let's get this party started!

# KETO 101

Keto is short for "ketogenic," a dietary pattern that emphasizes carb restriction paired with adequate intake of healthy fats and protein. Here's a brief refresher on the diet for those who need it.

## MACROS ARE KEY

Keto success revolves around eating an optimal balance of macronutrients, or "macros" for short: fat, protein, and carbs. Macros provide the energy content in our diets. Just like gas in a car, macros give the body fuel to function. In many traditional dietary patterns, carbohydrates supply the most fuel. The body runs on carbs and relies mainly on a sugar-burning metabolism. Keto is different. The diet limits carbs, pushing the body to rely primarily on fat for fuel. As a result, a metabolic shift known as ketosis occurs, effectively turning the body into a fat-burning machine.

Carbohydrates are reduced to a maximum daily total of 50 grams (20 to 30g net carbs) to support this change in metabolism, according to a review in *The American Journal of Clinical Nutrition*. Depending on how much you eat per day, 50 grams of carbohydrate can be between 4 and 19 percent of your total calories.

Keto is commonly described as low-carb, high-fat, moderate-protein, as is illustrated by the suggested proportions of macronutrients in the daily diet:

- **Carbs** (4 calories per gram): 4 to 19 percent of total calories

- **Protein** (4 calories per gram): 10 to 30 percent of total calories

- **Fat** (9 calories per gram): 60 to 90 percent of total calories

As you can see, these ranges are not terribly prescriptive. The actual proportions of macros in your diet will vary depending on your energy needs, body composition, and goals. The macro percentages of a competitive bodybuilder, for example, probably won't match the macros of a petite ballet dancer. Similarly, the macros needed for weight loss will be quite a bit different than those needed for therapeutic purposes. The truth is, this diet looks a little different for everyone.

To calculate macros that make sense for *your* body, visit the calculator tool on my website (Ketogasm.com/keto-calculator).

## WHAT'S KETOSIS?

Regardless of individual macro targets, the one common thread among keto dieters is cutting carbs to support ketosis. When you stop stoking the furnace with carbs, the body adapts to a more readily available fuel source: fat. Ketosis is the naturally occurring metabolic shift in which the body no longer burns sugar but uses fat for energy and the production of ketones. Ketones are another form of energy the body can use to replace glucose in the absence of carbohydrates.

Once you taper your carb intake, the body must burn through stored sugars before it fully ramps up ketone production. Getting into ketosis usually takes a few days of very low-carb eating (<50g carbs/day). However, body composition and physical activity can accelerate or slow down the process.

If you're just getting started with keto, ketone test strips can provide some insight into your state of ketosis. In the early days of ketosis, when your body isn't fully adapted to using fat as a fuel source, not all ketones are used up, and the excess ketones are eliminated in the urine. The strips measure the presence of those ketones.

Over time, as your fat-burning efficiency increases, your body wastes fewer ketones. When this happens, the test strips will fail to detect the presence of ketones—a "false negative" that misleads dieters into thinking that they are no longer in ketosis. A more accurate reading of ketone levels can be provided by ketone blood monitors and breathalyzers, but they can be a bit pricey.

Testing is optional for many people. If you'd rather not fuss with ketone levels and medical devices, trust the process and stick with delicious, keto-friendly food and beverages that fit your macros.

## STAYING IN KETOSIS WHILE DRINKING

Navigating food and drinks that support ketosis can be a little tricky at first, but rest assured, you can absolutely enjoy alcoholic beverages on keto once you know what to look for. By all means, if cocktails light you up, I encourage you to indulge when the mood strikes. The key to success with any dietary pattern is finding what works for you. Ask anyone who has successfully changed their eating habits, and they will share the same secret: It's not restriction and deprivation that drive success, it's sustainability. The all-or-nothing mindset will only get you so far. To that end, I encourage you to approach keto less like a rigid diet, and more like an adaptable lifestyle choice—booze included.

One surprising benefit of drinking alcohol on a low-carb diet is the cost savings. Keto lowers your alcohol tolerance, translating to less money spent at bars and liquor stores. Most keto dieters prefer to play home bartender, mixing creative concoctions to perfectly pair with their dietary needs for a fraction of the price.

Drinking on keto does have its challenges out in the wild. *What* and *how much* you drink will affect your ability to stay in ketosis. Unfortunately, most bars don't cater to the keto crowd, and many alcoholic beverages, mixers, and garnishes are locked and loaded with sugar. We'll explore which drinks best support ketosis to prep you for nights out on the town in just a bit (see page 6). But first, there are a few considerations to keep in mind about how alcohol affects the body on a low-carb diet.

**Booze counts toward your daily calorie and carb counts.** At about 7 calories per gram, alcohol provides energy and thus contributes to your daily calorie intake, similar to macronutrients. Although pure ethanol is carb-free, the sugars in alcoholic beverages and mixers do add to your carb tally.

**Alcohol delays fat-burning.** When you drink alcohol, your body temporarily shifts out of fat-burning mode to prioritize alcohol metabolism. In other words, your body presses pause on using energy (both from the food you eat and the fuel your body has stored) while it clears alcohol from your system.

**Ketosis lowers your alcohol tolerance, so you may be more of a lightweight.** It's important to practice moderation and pace yourself while drinking; ketosis amplifies the effects of alcohol. With lowered alcohol tolerance, be safe and play it cool—a little goes a long way!

**Beware of the munchies when drinking.** Lowered inhibition often leads to food decisions that you aren't proud of, but drunk-dialing food deliveries can be avoided with a little forethought. When the munchies set in, having low-carb food options available makes it much easier to stick to your game plan.

**Alcohol dehydrates you.** Alcohol has a diuretic effect, causing you to flush out water instead of retaining it. This leads to dehydration—and the dreaded hangover—if you don't replenish your body with water. A good rule of thumb is to drink one glass of water per drink, and another glass before bed. (For more hangover hacks, see the box on the next page.)

# HANGOVER HELP

With the altered metabolism of ketosis and lowered alcohol tolerance, keto hangovers can be especially vicious. Staying hydrated is essential for hangover prevention, but these tried and true strategies will help you recuperate if things get ugly.

**RESTORE ELECTROLYTES.** Good advice for any keto dieter, but especially the hungover one. As your body flushes out water, it's also quickly dumping sodium, potassium, and other water-soluble minerals and vitamins. Consider sugar-free sports drinks, multivitamins, or electrolyte supplements for relief.

**EAT UP.** Grab a bite to eat to give your body a nutrient boost and settle your stomach. The food recipes in chapters 12 and 13 are fair game for happy hour and hangovers alike.

**SLEEP IT OFF.** If you're partying all night, your body is robbed of critical repair time. Sleep is restorative, and one of the best ways to bounce back after a long night is to catch some Zs. Take a power nap or sleep in late.

**GET MOVING.** Exercise will help the natural detox process along and boost your mood. It might not be the best workout of your life, but you'll feel a lot better afterward.

# THE KETO ALCOHOL CHEAT SHEET

Now that you know how alcohol impacts low-carb dieting, it's time to learn what type of drinks you can enjoy on keto. You may be pleasantly surprised by the variety available to you right out of the gate. With a little keto mixology, the possibilities are endless.

## WINE

Relax, wine o'clock has not been canceled. But before you grab your favorite bottle of vino, it's important to note that the carbs in wine vary. The amount of residual sugar (that which is left over after fermentation) and the dosage of additional sugar used in the production of some wines, such as champagne, determines the final carb count. Avoid sweet fortified and dessert wines and go for dry varieties instead. Check the label for clues about sweetness. Champagnes and sparkling wines, for example, are classified by sugar content. From driest to sweetest, they are brut nature, extra brut, brut, extra-dry, sec, demi-sec, and doux. Serving size: 5 fluid ounces.

### REDS

| WINE | CARBS | CALORIES |
|---|---|---|
| Barbera | 4.1g | 125 |
| Burgundy | 5.5g | 127 |
| Cabernet Franc | 3.6g | 122 |
| Cabernet Sauvignon | 3.8g | 122 |
| Carignane | 3.5g | 109 |
| Claret | 4.4g | 122 |
| Gamay | 3.5g | 115 |
| Grenache | 3.8g | 122 |
| Lemberger | 3.6g | 118 |
| Malbec | 3.8g | 125 |
| Merlot | 3.7g | 122 |
| Mourvèdre | 3.9g | 129 |

| WINE | CARBS | CALORIES |
|---|---|---|
| Petite Sirah | 3.9g | 125 |
| Pinot Noir | 3.4g | 122 |
| Sangiovese | 3.9g | 126 |
| Syrah/Shiraz | 3.8g | 122 |
| Zinfandel | 4.2g | 129 |

## WHITES

| WINE | CARBS | CALORIES |
|---|---|---|
| Chardonnay | 3.2g | 123 |
| Chenin Blanc | 4.9g | 118 |
| Fumé Blanc | 3.3g | 121 |
| Gewürztraminer | 3.8g | 119 |
| Muscat/Moscato | 7.8g | 123 |
| Müller-Thurgau | 5.2g | 112 |
| Pinot Blanc | 2.9g | 119 |
| Pinot Gris/Grigio | 3.0g | 122 |
| Riesling | 5.5g | 118 |
| Sauvignon Blanc | 3.0g | 119 |
| Sémillon | 4.5g | 121 |

## SPARKLING WINES AND ROSÉ

| WINE | CARBS | CALORIES |
|---|---|---|
| Asti Spumante | 3.8g | 121 |
| Cava | 3.8g | 121 |
| Champagne | 3.8g | 121 |
| Prosecco | 3.8g | 121 |
| Rosé | 5.8g | 121 |
| Sparkling Wine | 3.8g | 121 |

## BEER AND HARD CIDER

Most traditional ciders and beers tend to be high in carbs. But thanks to the increasing popularity of keto, the number of craft brews proudly displaying low-carb labels has recently exploded. When in doubt, choose "light" beer. Serving size: 12 fluid ounces.

| BEER/CIDER | CARBS | CALORIES |
|---|---|---|
| Anyday Rosé Cider | 6.0g | 125 |
| Brewery Ommegang Brut IPA | 3.9g | 140 |
| Bridge Brewing Co. PrimeTime | 1.5g | 110 |
| Deschutes Brewery Da Shootz! Pilsner | 4.2g | 99 |
| Devil's Backbone Brewing Co. Bright Tangerine | 2.0g | 85 |
| Dogfish Head Slightly Mighty Lo-Cal IPA | 3.6g | 95 |
| Kona Brewing Co. Kanaha Blonde Ale | 4.0g | 99 |
| Lagunitas Daytime IPA | 3.0g | 98 |
| Pittsburgh Brewing Co. IC Light | 2.8g | 95 |
| Pittsburgh Brewing Co. IC Light Mango | 4.0g | 95 |
| R&D Brewing LoCal Resolution Ale | 2.4g | 98 |
| Saint Archer Brewing Co. Gold | 2.6g | 95 |
| Samuel Smith's Organic Cider | 2.9g | 178 |
| Shiner Light Blonde | 3.8g | 99 |
| Shiner Ruby Redbird | 3.1g | 95 |

## SPIRITS

Of all the boozy beverages, distilled spirits tend to be the easiest to navigate on keto. That's because most contain no carbs! Nada. Zip, zero, zilch. Vodka, whiskey, rum, gin, tequila, brandy—you name it, no carbs. *Flavored* spirits, on the other hand, do contain sugars. Avoid flavored liquors. As an alternative, consider crafting unique infusions with extracts, herbs, and fruits. See Mixers, Garnishes, and Flavors (page 10) and chapter 11 (page 115) for more options. Serving size: 1½ fluid ounces.

| SPIRIT | CARBS | CALORIES |
|---|---|---|
| Absinthe | 0g | 97 |
| Brandy/Cognac | 0g | 97 |
| Gin | 0g | 97 |
| Moonshine | 0g | 125 |
| Rum | 0g | 97 |
| Soju | 0g | 64 |
| Tequila/Mezcal | 0g | 97 |
| Vodka | 0g | 97 |
| Whiskey/Bourbon/Scotch | 0g | 97 |

## HARD SELTZERS/HARD LEMONADES/WINE COOLERS

It's best to steer clear of hard lemonades and wine coolers; the sugar in some of these drinks can put you over your carb limit for the entire day. Instead, grab a hard seltzer, which is great for casual hangs and backyard barbecues. With a wide range of flavors and only trace carbs, these sparkling waters also make fantastic cocktail mixers. Serving size: 12 fluid ounces.

| ALCOHOL | CARBS | CALORIES |
|---|---|---|
| Bon & Viv Spiked Seltzer | 2.0g | 90 |
| Henry's Hard Seltzer | 1.6g | 88 |
| Smirnoff Spiked Sparkling Seltzer | 1.0g | 90 |
| Truly Lemonade Hard Seltzer | 3.0g | 100 |
| Truly Hard Seltzer | 2.0g | 100 |
| White Claw Hard Seltzer | 2.0g | 100 |
| Wild Basin Boozy Sparkling Water | 1.0g | 100 |

# MIXERS, GARNISHES, AND FLAVORS

Keep an eye on sugar content. Most sodas, juices, sweet teas, tonics, syrups, and drink mixes land far outside the realm of keto compatibility. Stick with unsweetened, sugar-free, and diet options or get creative with DIY flavors. Chapter 11 has keto-fied versions of the most popular syrups and mixers to help you get started.

| MIXER/GARNISH/FLAVOR | CARBS | CALORIES |
|---|---|---|
| Bitters (Angostura, Peychaud's) | 0.3g | 13 (per teaspoon) |
| Club soda | 0g | 0 |
| Coffee | 0g | 1 (per cup) |
| Diet soda (Zevia, diet cola, diet ginger beer/ale) | 0g | 0 |
| Diet tonic water | 0g | 0 |
| Extracts (vanilla, peppermint, orange, almond, etc.) | <1.0g | 0–12 (per teaspoon) |
| Flavored waters (Bai, Hint, Sparkling Ice) | 0 | 0–10 |
| Fresh berries (blackberry, blueberry, strawberry) | 1.2–1.6g | 9–15 (per ounce) |
| Fresh herbs (mint, rosemary, basil) | <1.0g | 2.5 (per tablespoon) |
| Hot sauce (Tabasco, Sriracha, Tapatío) | 0–1g | 0–5 (per teaspoon) |
| Olives | 0.1g | 4.4 (per olive) |
| Pickles | 0.4g | 3.4 (per ounce) |
| Salt (coarse, kosher, or sea) | 0g | 0 |
| Seltzer | 0g | 0 |
| Sparkling water (La Croix, Bubly, Perrier, Waterloo, etc.) | 0g | 0 |
| Sugar-free juices (fresh squeezed citrus, diet cranberry juice) | <1.0–2.6g | 0.6–7.7 (per ounce) |
| Tomato juice | 1.1g | 5.2 (per ounce) |
| Unsweetened low-carb milks (heavy cream, coconut milk, almond milk) | 0–1g | 5–101 (per ounce) |
| Unsweetened tea | 0g | 0–3 (per cup) |
| Water flavorings: (H2wOw, Mio, Stur) | <1g | 0–3 |
| Worcestershire sauce | 1g | 5 (per teaspoon) |

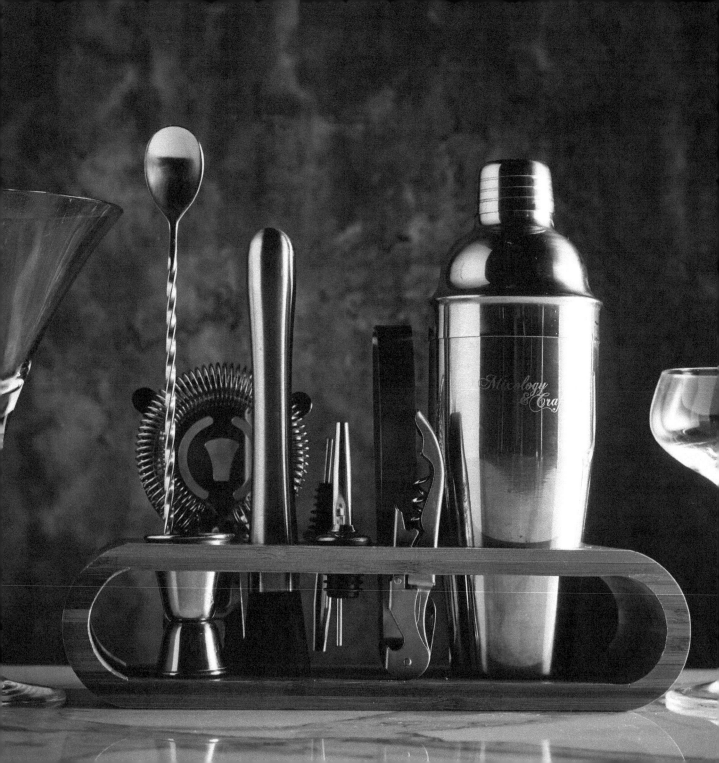

# = 2 =

# BUILDING YOUR LOW-CARB BAR

Now that you have a good idea about what kinds of ingredients are at your disposal, we can dive into the terms, tools, and steps that make a cocktail a *cocktail*. In this chapter, you'll learn the essentials for creating a practical home bar to make this book's recipes and many others.

# HOW TO SPEAK BARTENDER

When it comes to mixology, there's a distinct lingo that occurs behind the bar. Because you'll be the one mixing drinks, it's time to expand your cocktail vocabulary. The terms below will help you fine-tune your drink-building skills.

**Chaser:** A beverage you have immediately after drinking something with alcohol, typically a shot of liquor. Chasers suitable for keto include popular low-carb mixers (see page 10) and light beers (see page 8).

**Dash:** A unit of measurement that loosely translates to a few drops of an ingredient. Dasher tops are often used on bitters bottles to release the small volume, with one shake of the bottle yielding one dash.

**Dry:** A descriptive designation for wines that relates to the sweetness; *dry* roughly translates to "not sweet." The drier the better when it comes to keeping carbs low.

**Float:** A technique that involves slowly pouring a liquid ingredient over the surface of a drink to create a separate layer that appears to "float" on top without mixing. To achieve the effect, hover an upside-down spoon over the liquid in the glass and deliberately pour at a snail's pace, letting the liquid crawl down the back of the spoon and onto the drink.

**Mixer:** A nonalcoholic beverage, or one with lower alcohol by volume, added to a drink containing hard alcohol. Typically used to flavor or dilute spirits.

**Modifier:** An ingredient that alters and enhances the base spirit in a cocktail, and is often essential to the flavor and texture of the drink.

**Muddle:** A technique used to mash ingredients at the bottom of a glass with a tool. Fruits, herbs, and sweeteners are often muddled together, as seen in the recipes for the Bramble (page 55) and Mojito (Mo-Keto!) (page 75).

**Neat:** An individual spirit served at room temperature without ice, a chilled glass, or any additional ingredients.

**On the rocks:** A phrase to describe a drink served over ice.

**Shake:** A technique used to mix ingredients together by agitating a shaker tool. Shaking a drink serves multiple purposes beyond mixing, including chilling, dilution, aeration, and emulsification.

**Splash:** A nonstandard measurement to describe a small amount of liquid added to a cocktail, a volume anywhere between a dash and an ounce.

**Stir:** A technique used to mix ingredients together with a bar spoon.

**Straight:** A spirit served alone, without other liquor or mixers. It can be served in a chilled glass, over ice, and occasionally with a splash of water.

**Strain:** A technique used to keep ice and solid ingredients out of the finished drink by pouring the mixed cocktail through a strainer tool. Strained drinks can be served "up" or "on the rocks" with fresh ice.

**Top off:** To pour the last ingredient into a cocktail, filling the glass to the top.

**Up:** A phrase to describe a drink served without ice in the glass. The beverage is chilled by shaking or stirring with ice and then strained into a chilled glass.

# THE LIQUIDS

When stocking a home bar, practicality is where it's at. The following setup will allow you to make tasty keto cocktails any time you like. Start by stocking ingredients that speak to your tastes. The recipes in this book are organized by spirit, so you can readily find cocktails that make use of what you have on hand.

## ESSENTIAL INGREDIENTS

### LIQUORS

Choose unflavored, distilled spirits to avoid high carb counts. Because of their distillation methods, the "top-shelf" liquors tend to have less of a "burn" going down. The budget-friendly spirits are harsher on the palate but are equal as far as carbs go.

Whiskey/whisky (bourbon, Scotch, rye): These alcohols are grain-based (corn, barley, rye, or wheat) and aged in oak casks. The type of grain and the location in which the spirit is made determine the whiskey category. For example, bourbon is made with corn in the United States, barley-based Scotch comes from Scotland, and rye is produced in the United States and Canada from rye (a grass similar to wheat).

Brandy: Brandy is distilled from fermented fruit juice or wine, produced from grapes and other fruits. Cognac is a type of brandy made using white grapes from the Cognac region in France.

Gin: Gin is distilled from grain with botanicals, most commonly juniper berries.

Rum (silver, light, dark): Rum is distilled from fermented sugarcane juice or sugarcane molasses and often aged in oak barrels.

Tequila and mezcal: Tequila is distilled from the blue agave plant in Mexico, whereas mezcal is produced from various agave plants in the same region. Though tequila is technically a mezcal, it lacks the signature smoky flavor (and the infamous worm in the bottle).

Vodka: Vodka is distilled from grain or vegetables, such as potatoes.

## LIQUEUR SUBSTITUTES

Liqueurs are spirits that are sweetened or flavored. The following (both homemade and store-bought) are suitable replacements on keto.

- Cherry water flavoring (maraschino substitute)
- Homemade Amaretto (page 119)
- Low-Carb Coffee Liqueur (page 118)
- Low-Carb Orange Liqueur (page 117)
- Pomegranate water flavoring (grenadine substitute)

- Unsweetened flavor extracts or concentrates, including vanilla, chocolate, mint, orange, cherry, honey, etc.
- Unsweetened pomegranate juice (Campari substitute)

## SUGAR ALTERNATIVES

Satisfy your sweet tooth without adding carbs. These sweeteners do not directly impact ketosis and therefore get subtracted from total carbs when calculating "net carbs" (as you do with fiber).

**Allulose:** A nonmetabolizing form of sugar that tastes nearly identical to the real deal with no aftertaste. It quickly dissolves in liquids and functions as you would expect sugar to do in recipes, making it perfect for cocktails and syrups. It comes in crystallized and powdered forms.

**Erythritol:** A sugar alcohol that is slightly less sweet than sugar. A mint-like cooling effect and aftertaste is noticeable in large quantities, but won't affect your cocktails. It comes in granular, powdered, and brown sugar forms.

**Monk fruit:** A plant-based sweetener with no aftertaste, made from melon. It is potently sweet, much more so than sugar. To balance this, brands often blend monk fruit with erythritol or allulose.

**Stevia:** A sweetener made from the leaves of the stevia plant, far sweeter than sugar with an occasional bitter aftertaste. Stevia comes in liquid and powdered forms, but look out for high-carb bulking agents (e.g., dextrose, maltodextrin, etc.) used in some powders.

The recipes in this book call for specific sweeteners and amounts, but can easily be adapted to a sweetener of your choice using the following conversions:*

1 teaspoon sugar = 1¼ teaspoons allulose = 1¼ teaspoons erythritol = 1 teaspoon monk fruit blend = 1 pinch pure monk fruit = 1 to 2 drops liquid stevia = 1 pinch powdered stevia leaf extract

*Conversions may vary by brand and specific blends. Check the ingredient list and packaging label for guidance.

# COCKTAIL CONSTRUCTION

Once you learn the "anatomy" of a drink, navigating the world of cocktails becomes a breeze. You'll be developing winning flavor combinations and recipes in no time. Building new cocktails can be just as fun as drinking them! Here's a cheat sheet to get you started:

**THE BASE:** The main alcohol component the drink is built upon. Layers of flavor, texture, and aroma are added to this foundation. Spirits are considered the base for most cocktails.

**THE BODY:** Also known as the "modifier." This element transforms a spirit into an actual cocktail, enhancing the liquor without overpowering it. The body changes the flavor, texture, and consistency while tying each ingredient together. Mixers, liqueurs, and even ice often serve this purpose.

**THE PERFUME:** The smallest component of the drink, used to highlight the base and balance the cocktail by adding a complementary hint of flavor, an aromatic element, or a splash of color. Syrups, fruits, herbs, and garnishes fall into this category.

# THE GLASSES

Although there is an endless variety of cocktail glassware with specific purposes, serving a drink in the "wrong" glass is by no means a deal-breaker. However, presentation is an integral part of the cocktail experience, so being resourceful is essential when it comes to bartending at home. Only have red plastic cups? Serve that drink with confidence and pride! But if you would like to take it up a notch, these are the most functional glasses you need to get you started.

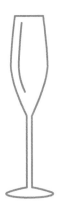  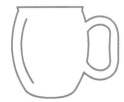

**Champagne flute:** These tulip-shaped, long-stemmed glasses (6 to 9 ounces) are tall and narrow to keep the bubbles flowing in fizzy champagne and sparkling wines, as seen in the French Kiss (page 35) and Champagne Cocktail (page 33).

**Cocktail/Coupe:** These long-stemmed glasses (3 to 6 ounces) have shallow bowls that are ideal for sipping strained cocktails and smaller-size drinks, like the Vesper Martini (page 48) and Dirty Martini (page 85).

**Copper mug:** These metal mugs (16 to 20 ounces) insulate the temperature of cocktails chilled with ice and are traditionally used for the Moscow Mule (page 84).

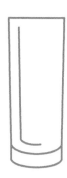

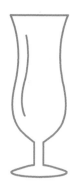

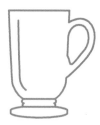

**Highball/Collins:** These tall, narrow glasses (10 to 16 ounces) work well for drinks served over ice and those with larger volumes, such as the Bramble (page 55) and Blackjack (page 38).

**Hurricane:** These curvy, short-stemmed glasses (16 to 20 ounces) are excellent for large frozen and tropical drinks, like the Piña Colada (page 72) and Bahama Mama (page 74).

**Irish coffee mug:** Made of thick, heatproof glass, these short-stemmed mugs (8 to 10 ounces) come equipped with handles to safely enjoy warm drinks, like Irish Coffee (page 100).

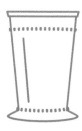

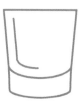

**Julep:** These metal cups (8 to 12 ounces) are typically made of silver and perfect for keeping drinks icy cold in warm weather, traditionally used for the Mint Julep (page 95).

**Rocks/old-fashioned:** Short and stout with a sturdy bottom, these tumblers (4 to 8 ounces) suit medium-volume drinks served over ice, like the Old-Fashioned (page 96) or Gin and Tonic (page 50), and can withstand muddling ingredients together.

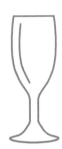

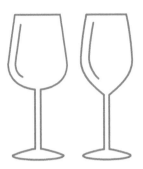

**Shot glass:** A small glass (1½ ounces) used for shots, shooters, and replacing the jigger measuring tool.

**Sour:** These tulip-shaped, short-stemmed glasses (5 to 6 ounces) are traditionally used for all varieties of sours, including the Pisco Sour (page 43) and Whiskey Sour (page 102).

**Wine glass:** These long-stemmed glasses (6 to 14 ounces) have deep, wide bowls that benefit swirling wine and can replace both cocktail and highball glasses if needed. A wine glass is the default for wine-based drinks, such as Sangria (page 34) and White Wine Spritzers (page 29).

# THE TOOLS

Mixing drinks without the right bartending tools is way harder than it has to be. You don't need to splurge on anything fancy; the basics are found in most budget-friendly bar kits. Below are the tools to get you started, as well as ways to repurpose your kitchenware as stand-ins in a pinch.

**Bar spoon:** Spoons with thin, extended handles to stir drinks and approximate teaspoon measurements. If you don't have a bar spoon, use a butter knife or thick straw to stir.

**Citrus squeezer/extractor:** A handheld press to juice lemons, limes, and oranges.

**Cocktail shaker:** A large, stainless steel cup (16 to 28 ounces) with a fitted top used to chill, shake, and pour drinks.

**Corkscrew:** A tool with a sturdy, metal spiral to remove corks from necks of bottles.

**Hawthorne strainer:** A flat handheld sieve with small holes and a coil of metal on its underside. The tool fits on top of a mixing glass or shaker and restrains the ice and solids when the drink is poured through the strainer into a glass. If you don't have one handy, you can strain your drinks with a slotted spoon.

**Jigger:** A measuring tool to portion approximately 1½ ounces for cocktails. A "jigger" is also a measurement itself, used instead of ounces in many cocktail recipes.

**Measuring spoons:** Spoons ranging from ¼ teaspoon to 1 tablespoon, making them perfect for measuring small volumes.

**Mixing glass:** A large, heavy-bottomed glass (16 to 20 ounces) used exclusively for mixing drinks rather than serving. If you don't have a mixing glass, a protein shaker cup or French press coffee carafe can come in handy.

**Muddler:** A long, blunt tool to crush, grind, and mix ingredients at the bottom of a mixing glass, much like the pestle in a mortar. If you don't have a muddler, you can use a wooden spoon.

**Paring knife:** A tiny knife that's handy for slicing and dicing citrus, herbs, and ginger.

# FINISHING TOUCHES

A cleverly chosen garnish can elevate any cocktail with rich aromas, flavors, and visual appeal. Consider upgrading your mixed drinks with one of the following techniques for a grand finale.

**MAKE A CITRUS TWIST OR SPIRAL GARNISH.** Use a sharp paring knife, vegetable peelér, or citrus stripper to cut strips of citrus peel. For a twist, cut off a wide 2-inch-long section. Holding the peel above the drink, zest-side down, twist it to release the oils, then run it along the rim of the glass and pop it into the drink. For a spiral, cut a long, thin strip, starting from one side of the fruit, working in a circular pattern. Wrap the peel around your finger to set the coil before garnishing the cocktail.

**FLAME A PEEL.** A sure-fire way to impress your guests, flaming a peel involves expressing citrus oil over a lit match so it briefly catches fire. Cut a wide round (1 to 2 inches in diameter) from the peel of fresh citrus. Light a match and hold it over the cocktail. With your other hand, position the round of peel above the flame, zest-side down. Give the piece of peel a quick squeeze between your fingers to release and ignite the oils. Wipe the rim of the glass with the peel and serve it in the drink.

**RIM A GLASS WITH CITRUS.** Slice a wedge from a lemon, lime, orange, or grapefruit. Swipe the fruit around the rim of the glass to leave traces of fruit juice where you sip.

**CREATE A SUGAR OR SALT RIM.** Once you've glazed the edge of the glass with citrus, you can take it a step further by dipping it in sugar or salt. Of course, traditional sugar can be swapped with keto-compatible sweeteners to keep the carbs low. I recommend using crystallized allulose for this purpose, but feel free to experiment. Although kosher salt is the most popular for salt rims, sea salt and Himalayan pink salt also work well.

**"SPANK" HERBS.** Activate the aromatic oils in your herbal garnishes by giving them a quick clap between your hands. Slide the "naughty" herb sprig in the drink and enjoy.

**FLOAT HERBS.** Similar to the carefully poured, unmixed top layer of the liquid float (see page 14), placing herbs on the surface of the drink or draped over the glass instead of mixing them in has a striking visual impact.

# ABOUT THE RECIPES

The upcoming cocktail chapters are sorted by spirit, so you can zip straight to your favorites and get started. Though many of the recipes are inspired by classics, they are by no means traditional. My goal is not to offend cocktail purists, but to help you build similar low-carb flavors, which can't always be done with conventional ingredients. For your convenience, each recipe has a Net Carb label listed right at the top. Every drink also includes tips and variations to help you keep the carbs low and put a different spin on recipes that play well with other flavors. Each recipe yields one drink, unless otherwise noted.

The recipes were developed to provide a wide range of drink options while keeping the number of ingredients purchased within reason. That means you'll be able to make the drinks from your home bar instead of going on a wild goose chase to hunt for obscure potions. Most of the ingredients included here are ready and waiting at your local grocery or liquor store. The baking aisle is your best bet for finding specialty items (such as sweeteners, low-carb flours, xanthan gum thickener/stabilizer, and certain extracts). However, some things may be easier to order through online retailers.

After the beverage chapters, you'll find a balanced assortment of keto appetizers, snacks, pub fare, and desserts to delight your guests while entertaining (see chapters 12 and 13). For those with allergies or dietary restrictions, dairy-free, gluten-free, nut-free, and vegan or vegetarian labels are included.

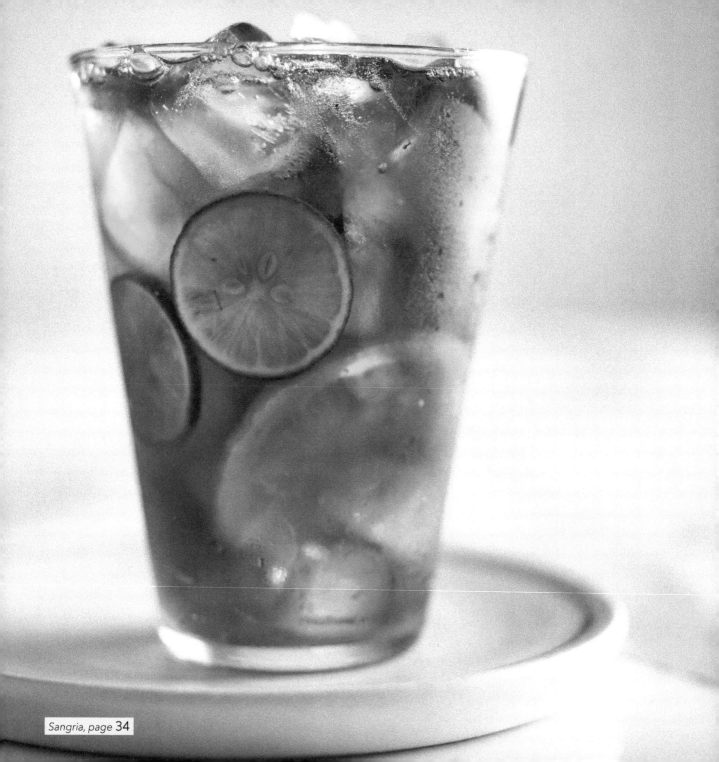

*Sangria, page* **34**

# = 3 =

# BEER, CHAMPAGNE, AND WINE COCKTAILS

# ALE FLIP

The ale flip can be a polarizing drink—you either love it or hate it. After reading through the recipe, you'll have a pretty good sense of what side of the fence you're on. If the thought of drinking a frothy warm dessert beer entices you, you're in for a real treat. Many of the cocktails we know today were invented during Prohibition, but this drink is even *more* old-school—think before refrigerators and ice machines.

8 ounces R&D Brewing LoCal Resolution Ale or low-carb beer of choice

½ ounce freshly squeezed lemon juice

1½ ounces brandy

1 ounce Low-Carb Simple Syrup (page 116)

1 large egg yolk

Nutmeg, ground or grated, for garnish

TOOLS: saucepan, citrus squeezer, jigger, medium bowl, whisk, beer mug, bar spoon

Heat the ale and lemon juice in a saucepan over medium-low heat until steam rises, then remove from the heat. In a medium bowl, whisk together the brandy, simple syrup, and egg yolk. Continue whisking and slowly add 2 ounces of the heated ale to the egg mixture, beating until smooth. Transfer the mixture to a mug, then carefully fill with the remaining warm beer and stir. Serve garnished with nutmeg.

PREP TIP: To make your drink as thick and frothy as can be, transfer the mixture back and forth between the saucepan and a pitcher several times before serving.

PER SERVING: CALORIES: 220; TOTAL FAT: 5G; TOTAL CARBOHYDRATES: 4G; FIBER: 0G; PROTEIN: 3G; SUGAR: 0G; SWEETENER CARBS: 16G

# WHITE WINE SPRITZER

The beauty of a wine spritzer is that even though the drink is simplicity itself, people are still impressed by it. The secret is to serve the spritzer icy cold, so be sure to chill the liquids thoroughly before mixing them. And if you'd rather be mingling with friends instead of showing off behind the bar, whip up a big batch of spritzers.

5 ounces pinot grigio or any dry white wine, chilled

3 ounces club soda, chilled

Lemon or orange twist, for garnish

TOOLS: wine glass, bar spoon, paring knife

Fill a wine glass with ice. Pour in the wine and club soda and delicately stir. Finish with a citrus twist.

MAKE IT A MOCKTAIL: Spritzers are always refreshing and can even be enjoyed booze-free. Nonalcoholic chardonnay is fantastic in this recipe.

PER SERVING: CALORIES: 122; TOTAL FAT: 0G; TOTAL CARBOHYDRATES: 3G; FIBER: 0G; PROTEIN: 0G; SUGAR: 0G; SWEETENER CARBS: 0G

# MICHELADA

This popular beer-based beverage is served throughout Latin America. Endless variations exist, but the most common recipes feature a salt-rimmed Mexican cerveza mixed with lime and hot sauce. Corona, Tecate, Modelo, Dos Equis, and Pacifico beers are frequently used in traditional Micheladas. However, you can use any low-carb beer you fancy.

Kosher salt, for garnish

Tajín Clasico seasoning, for garnish

Lime wedge

2 dashes Tabasco sauce or any hot sauce

Pinch freshly ground black pepper

12 ounces Corona Premier beer or low-carb beer of choice, chilled

TOOLS: small plate, paring knife, beer mug (chilled), bar spoon

On a small plate, mix the salt with the Tajín seasoning in a 1:1 ratio. Moisten the rim of a beer mug with the lime and dip the rim into the mixture. Fill the mug with ice and squeeze the lime juice into the glass. Add the hot sauce and black pepper, then slowly pour in the beer. Mix gently and serve with the lime wedge used for squeezing.

VARIATION: If you prefer a drink with more of a bite, trade the lime, hot sauce, and black pepper for a squeeze of fresh lemon juice and a shot of tequila. Feel free to omit the Tajín, hot sauce, and black pepper if fiery flavors aren't your thing—you'll still have a Michelada!

PER SERVING: CALORIES: 110; TOTAL FAT: 0G; TOTAL CARBOHYDRATES: 2G; FIBER: 0G; PROTEIN: 0G; SUGAR: 0G; SWEETENER CARBS: 0G

# FROSÉ SLUSHIE

**MAKES 5 DRINKS**

When the weather heats up, an icy slushie is a great way to cool down. Wine slushies are a playful way to enjoy your vino, and the novelty never wears off. Seriously, your guests will love you! These frozen cocktails are perfect for a hot summer day, but chances are you'll want to enjoy this recipe year-round.

4 cups ice

12 ounces rosé wine, chilled

½ cup frozen strawberries

TOOLS: blender, wine glass (chilled)

Add the ice, rosé, and strawberries to a blender. Blend until smooth and serve in wine glasses.

VARIATION: As far as low-carb wines go, rosé sits on the higher end of the carb spectrum. To further reduce the sugars in this recipe, make your slushies with a dry white wine and consider flavoring with fruit extracts instead of fresh fruit.

**PER SERVING:** CALORIES: 64; TOTAL FAT: 0G; TOTAL CARBOHYDRATES: 5G; FIBER: 0G; PROTEIN: 0G; SUGAR: 0G; SWEETENER CARBS: 0G

# RED WINE COOLER

Store-bought wine coolers are notoriously high in carbs. But this recipe delivers all the flavor and then some, with a fraction of the sugar. Given its relatively low alcohol content, this cocktail is terrific for casual social sipping.

6 ounces cabernet sauvignon or dry red wine of choice, chilled

4 ounces diet lemon-lime soda, chilled

Lemon or lime twist, for garnish

TOOLS: highball glass, bar spoon, paring knife

Fill a glass halfway with ice. Pour in the wine and soda and stir until blended. Garnish with a citrus twist.

> VARIATION: If you prefer white wine over red, swap out the cabernet sauvignon for a dry white. Chardonnay, pinot blanc, pinot gris, and sauvignon blanc are all great low-carb options for a white wine cooler.

PER SERVING: CALORIES: 147; TOTAL FAT: 0G; TOTAL CARBOHYDRATES: 5G; FIBER: 0G; PROTEIN: 0G; SUGAR: 0G; SWEETENER CARBS: 0G

# CHAMPAGNE COCKTAIL

This keto twist on the classic champagne cocktail transforms an inexpensive bottle of bubbly into something worthy of any celebration. Choose dry, low-sugar varieties of champagne and replace the traditional sugar cubes with keto-friendly sweetener to achieve the same flavor profile but with fewer carbs. Whether for poppin' bottles with friends or making a romantic toast by candlelight, this cocktail is sure to be a hit.

½ teaspoon monk fruit blend with erythritol or sweetener of choice

2 dashes Angostura bitters

4 ounces brut, extra brut, or brut nature champagne

Lemon twist, for garnish

TOOLS: champagne flute (chilled), paring knife

Place the monk fruit sweetener at the bottom of a champagne flute and soak the sweetener with the Angostura bitters. Fill the glass with champagne and garnish with a lemon twist.

PREP TIP: Champagne carb content varies by type, depending on the amount of sugar used in production. The following types of champagne have less than 3g carbs per 5-ounce serving: extra dry, brut, extra brut, brut nature, pas dosé, and dosage zéro ("Dosage, or 'Liqueur D'expédition,'" n.d., in the References on page 172). Avoid higher-carb champagnes, including sec, demi-sec, and doux.

PER SERVING: CALORIES: 97; TOTAL FAT: 0G; TOTAL CARBOHYDRATES: 3G; FIBER: 0G; PROTEIN: 0G; SUGAR: 1G; SWEETENER CARBS: 0G

NET CARBS
**2**G
PER DRINK

# SANGRIA

**MAKES 10 DRINKS**

Because sangria is made in big batches instead of single servings, it's ideal for parties and gatherings, which is great, because this cocktail is a huge crowd-pleaser. Though sangria is traditionally made with lots of chopped and muddled fruit, I've scaled back those ingredients to reduce the carbs. Be sure to account for the chilling time in your prep plans.

1 lemon, sliced

1 lime, sliced

1 (750 ml) bottle merlot or any dry red wine, chilled

1½ ounces brandy

1 ounce Low-Carb Orange Liqueur (page 117)

12 ounces club soda, chilled

**TOOLS:** large punch bowl or pitcher, jigger, wine glasses

Place the citrus slices in a punch bowl or pitcher. Add the wine, brandy, and orange liqueur, then stir to combine. Refrigerate for at least 2 hours or overnight. When ready to serve, stir in the club soda. Pour into ice-filled glasses to serve.

**VARIATION:** Sangria isn't limited to red wine: Dry white or rosé would be equally delightful. Herbs and berries also make wonderful choices in lieu of citrus. Raspberries, blackberries, strawberries, spearmint, or rosemary are all good options.

**PER SERVING:** CALORIES: 71; TOTAL FAT: 0G; TOTAL CARBOHYDRATES: 2G; FIBER: 0G; PROTEIN: 0G; SUGAR: 0G; SWEETENER CARBS: 0G

# FRENCH KISS

Known for its delicate rosy hue, effervescence, and raspberry notes, this drink will delight your guests as much by its elegance as by its flavor. Serve the eye-catching cocktail for special occasions and celebrations when toasts are made, such as Valentine's Day, New Year's Eve, bridal showers, and anniversaries.

8 raspberries, divided

1 ounce diet ginger beer, chilled

1 dash brandy

4 ounces brut or extra-brut champagne, chilled

TOOLS: mixing glass, muddler, jigger, champagne flute (chilled)

Place 6 raspberries in the bottom of a mixing glass. Add the ginger beer and brandy and muddle until the raspberries are completely mashed. Pour into a champagne flute and top with the champagne. Float the remaining 2 raspberries on the surface of the drink for garnish.

VARIATION: There's nothing like a little bubbly to celebrate the summer berry harvests. Consider swapping out the raspberries to change the color and flavor profile of the drink. Strawberries, blackberries, blueberries, and huckleberries are all excellent exchanges.

PER SERVING: CALORIES: 119; TOTAL FAT: 0G; TOTAL CARBOHYDRATES: 5G; FIBER: 1G; PROTEIN: 0G; SUGAR: 3G; SWEETENER CARBS: 0G

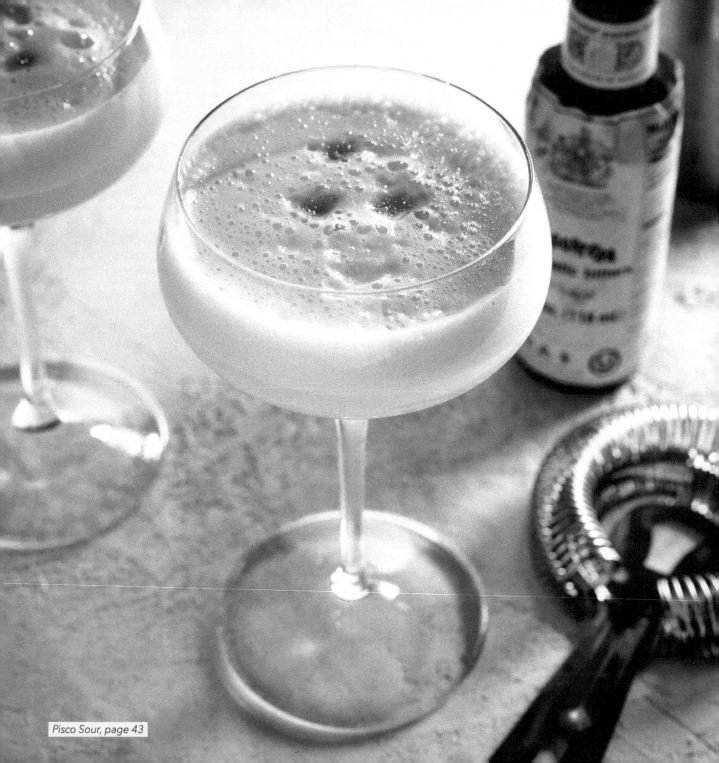

*Pisco Sour, page 43*

# = 4 =
# BRANDY

# BLACKJACK

Strong morning coffee or a stiff happy hour drink? Why choose when you can have the best of both worlds? Instead of kirsch (cherry brandy), plain brandy is used with sugar-free cherry flavoring to keto-fy this drink. This recipe is written to serve the cocktail icy cold, but you can easily make it a hot drink for nippy days by skipping the ice and using standard drip coffee.

2 ounces brandy

1½ ounces unsweetened cold brew coffee

½ teaspoon cherry water flavoring

Lemon twist, for garnish

TOOLS: highball glass, shaker, jigger, paring knife

Fill a glass with ice. Fill a shaker with ice and add the brandy, coffee, and cherry flavoring. Shake well and strain into the glass. Garnish with a lemon twist.

PREP TIP: When cold brew coffee is unavailable, hot brewed coffee is a fair swap. Just be sure to chill it first to prevent the ice from melting too quickly if you're serving the recipe as a cold drink.

PER SERVING: CALORIES: 129; TOTAL FAT: 0G; TOTAL CARBOHYDRATES: 0G; FIBER: 0G; PROTEIN: 0G; SUGAR: 0G; SWEETENER CARBS: 0G

# CHERRY BLOSSOM

Cherry cocktail flavors can be challenging to accomplish without racking up carbs. Sugar-free flavorings must be used in place of the kirsch and high-sugar maraschino cherries in the original. In this recipe, cherry water flavoring delivers the tart, cherry kick, but unsweetened extracts and flavored concentrates can yield similar results.

2 ounces brandy

½ ounce Low-Carb Orange Liqueur (page 117)

½ ounce freshly squeezed lemon juice

½ teaspoon cherry water flavoring

1 dash pomegranate water flavoring

TOOLS: shaker, jigger, citrus squeezer, strainer, cocktail glass (chilled)

Fill a shaker with ice and add the brandy, orange liqueur, lemon juice, cherry flavoring, and pomegranate flavoring and mix well. Strain into a glass.

VARIATION: Though this drink is traditionally made with brandy, bourbon is an excellent substitute spirit in this recipe. Unsweetened pomegranate juice can replace the pomegranate water flavoring if needed.

PER SERVING: CALORIES: 136; TOTAL FAT: 0G; TOTAL CARBOHYDRATES: 1G; FIBER: 0G; PROTEIN: 0G; SUGAR: 0G; SWEETENER CARBS: 3G

# BRANDY ALEXANDER

If you're a fan of dessert-like drinks, look no further—this drink is sinful decadence served in a glass. Dark crème de cacao liqueur is a staple in the traditional cocktail, but that syrupy-sweet ingredient drives the carb content up. Not a problem. Mix a little bit of cream, cacao, and vanilla extract with a low-carb simple syrup.

2 ounces Cognac or unflavored brandy of choice

1½ ounces heavy (whipping) cream

½ ounce Low-Carb Simple Syrup (page 116)

¼ teaspoon unsweetened cacao or cocoa powder

⅛ teaspoon vanilla extract

Nutmeg, grated or ground, for garnish

TOOLS: shaker, jigger, strainer, cocktail glass (chilled)

Fill a shaker with ice and add the Cognac, cream, simple syrup, cacao powder, and vanilla. Shake well and strain into a glass. Garnish with nutmeg.

VARIATION: If you don't have powdered cacao or cocoa on hand, chocolate extract is another option—just reduce the volume to ⅛ teaspoon.

PER SERVING: CALORIES: 278; TOTAL FAT: 16G; TOTAL CARBOHYDRATES: 2G; FIBER: 0G; PROTEIN: 1G; SUGAR: 1G; SWEETENER CARBS: 8G

# JACK ROSE

Unconventional keto-friendly substitutes are used in this recipe to capture the flavors of this classic cocktail while keeping carbs in check. Applejack, a carb-loaded apple brandy, is replaced with a combination of unflavored grape brandy and sugar-free apple flavoring, and grenadine is traded for pomegranate water flavoring.

2 ounces brandy

¾ ounce freshly squeezed lemon juice

1 or 2 drops pomegranate water flavoring

1 or 2 drops unsweetened apple liquid concentrate, extract, or water flavoring

1 dash Peychaud's bitters

Lemon twist, for garnish

TOOLS: shaker, jigger, citrus squeezer, strainer, cocktail glass (chilled), paring knife

Fill a shaker with ice and add the brandy, lemon juice, pomegranate water, apple flavoring, and bitters and shake well. Strain into a glass. Twist the lemon over the drink, wipe the rim with the lemon, and drop it into the glass.

VARIATION: Peychaud's bitters may be swapped for Angostura bitters, or any other bitters you may have on hand. The effect will be similar, though the spices in each will subtly alter the taste. If needed, unsweetened pomegranate juice can replace the pomegranate water flavoring.

PER SERVING: CALORIES: 134; TOTAL FAT: 0G; TOTAL CARBOHYDRATES: 1G; FIBER: 0G; PROTEIN: 0G; SUGAR: 1G; SWEETENER CARBS: 0G

# SIDECAR

This classic brandy sour highlights the robust, spicy Cognac base with the perfect sweet-to-tart ratio. Traditionally built with high-carb Cointreau, this recipe puts low-carb orange liqueur to work in its place. And of course, the sugar rim is anything but . . . instead, crystallized allulose sweetens the lip, though you can omit the garnish if you prefer.

Lemon wedge, for garnish (optional)

Crystallized allulose or sweetener of choice, for garnish (optional)

1½ ounces Cognac or unflavored brandy

¾ ounce Low-Carb Orange Liqueur (page 117)

¾ ounce freshly squeezed lemon juice

Lemon twist, for garnish

TOOLS: paring knife, small plate, cocktail glass (chilled), jigger, citrus squeezer, shaker, strainer

If desired, rim a glass: Moisten the rim of a glass with the lemon and dip the rim into the allulose; set aside. Fill a shaker with ice and add the Cognac, orange liqueur, and lemon juice and shake well. Strain into the glass and garnish with a lemon twist.

> VARIATION: Make it a Boston Sidecar by switching the lemons for limes and adding a shot of white or silver rum.

PER SERVING: CALORIES: 138; TOTAL FAT: 0G; TOTAL CARBOHYDRATES: 1G; FIBER: 0G; PROTEIN: 0G; SUGAR: 1G; SWEETENER CARBS: 4G

# PISCO SOUR

This classic cocktail is made with pisco, a grape brandy with a distinct, light, and fruity taste—unlike the spicy, bitter flavors found in other brandies, such as Cognac. When mixed with a bit of citrus, sweetener, and egg whites? Two words: frothy perfection.

2 ounces pisco brandy

1 ounce freshly squeezed lemon juice

½ ounce Low-Carb Simple Syrup (page 116)

1 large egg white

1 dash Angostura bitters

TOOLS: shaker, jigger, strainer, citrus squeezer, sour glass or cocktail glass (chilled)

Combine the pisco, lemon juice, simple syrup, and egg white in a shaker. Shake vigorously for at least 30 seconds. Add ice and shake again. Strain into a glass and carefully decorate the foam surface with a drop of bitters to garnish.

PREP TIP: For best results, be sure to do the double shake, once without ice and once with. Shaking ingredients without ice is called a "dry shake." When you do this with egg whites, the technique fully incorporates the components and at the same time aerates the egg protein. The shaken egg whites give the drink its thick foam, and dry shaking it first yields a more uniform, frothy texture. (If using raw egg whites is out of your comfort zone, consider opting for powdered egg whites instead to achieve the same airy, whipped consistency.)

PER SERVING: CALORIES: 129; TOTAL FAT: 0G; TOTAL CARBOHYDRATES: 2G; FIBER: 0G; PROTEIN: 4G; SUGAR: 1G; SWEETENER CARBS: 8G

# CORPSE REVIVER

This aptly named cocktail was initially developed to ward off hangovers, to be enjoyed the morning after a long night of drinking, in pure "hair of the dog that bit you" fashion. Traditionally made with sweet vermouth and applejack or Calvados, we opt for dry vermouth, apple flavoring, and sweetener to pull off the flavors.

1½ ounces brandy

¾ ounce dry vermouth

1 teaspoon crystallized allulose or sweetener of choice

1 or 2 drops unsweetened apple flavor liquid concentrate, extract, or water flavoring

TOOLS: mixing glass, bar spoon, jigger, strainer, cocktail glass (chilled)

Fill a mixing glass with ice and add the brandy, vermouth, allulose, and apple flavoring. Stir well and strain into a glass.

PREP TIP: Apple-flavored liquid concentrate may be a challenge to find while you're out grocery shopping, but online retailers carry the ingredient, as well as many big-box retailers. Liquid concentrates and extracts can be a great way to flavor spirits without the added carbs. They are also much more budget-friendly than stocking your bar with a variety of flavored spirits. Liquid water flavorings, like MiO, work great, too!

PER SERVING: CALORIES: 131; TOTAL FAT: 0G; TOTAL CARBOHYDRATES: 3G; FIBER: 0G; PROTEIN: 0G; SUGAR: 0G; SWEETENER CARBS: 0G

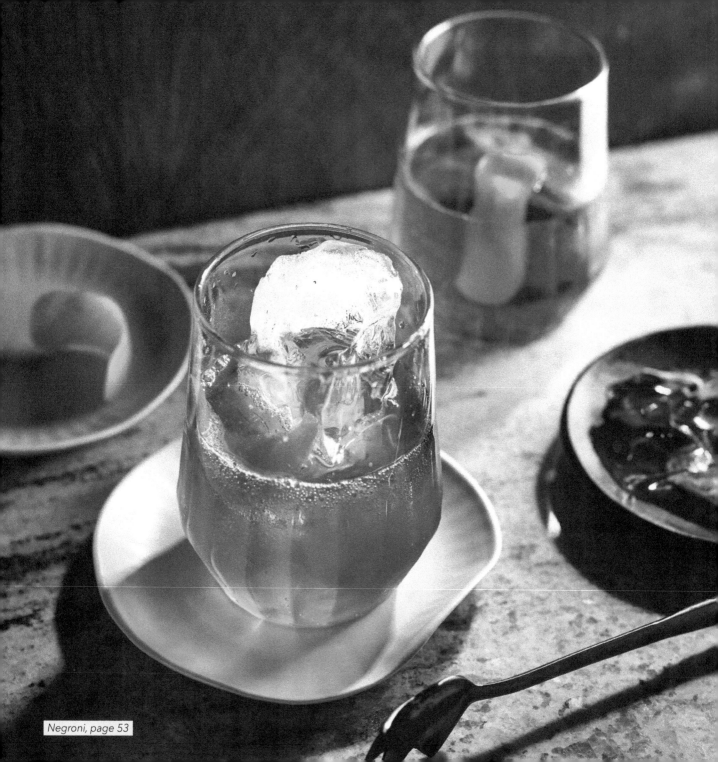

*Negroni, page 53*

# = 5 =

## GIN

# VESPER MARTINI

Don't you dare stir this drink! Secret agent James Bond invented the Vesper Martini. It should be enjoyed just as he intended: shaken, not stirred. Given the namesake of the original Bond girl, Vesper Lynd, this cocktail has become an iconic variation on the classic martini. Kina Lillet is the fortified wine traditionally used in the cocktail, though it's no longer available. Dry white wine has replaced it here to keep carbs low.

2 ounces gin

⅓ ounce sauvignon blanc or dry white wine of choice

¼ ounce vodka

Lemon twist, for garnish

**TOOLS:** shaker, jigger, strainer, cocktail glass (chilled), paring knife

Fill a shaker with ice and add the gin, wine, and vodka. Shake vigorously and strain into a glass. Twist the lemon over the drink, wipe the rim with the lemon, and drop it into the glass.

**VARIATION:** If you prefer to stick with a more classic drink in true Bond fashion, Lillet Blanc is an acceptable replacement for the wine in this recipe. Though the fortified wine has a higher carb content, the small amount called for keeps the carbs in check. Alternatively, dry vermouth may be used.

**PER SERVING:** CALORIES: 153; TOTAL FAT: 0G; TOTAL CARBOHYDRATES: 0G; FIBER: 0G; PROTEIN: 0G; SUGAR: 0G; SWEETENER CARBS: 0G

# DRAGONFLY

Similar to a Gin and Tonic (page 50), this cocktail features the sharp, spicy zing of ginger beer in place of the tonic, putting it in a league of its own. As ginger beer and ginger ale are both high-carb beverages, you'll need to opt for the diet versions of each to stay in the low-carb range. This drink is excellent year-round, but sipping one outdoors in warm weather as dragonflies zip around the garden is an otherworldly experience.

2 ounces gin

5 ounces diet ginger ale or diet ginger beer

Lime wedge, for garnish

TOOLS: highball glass, jigger, bar spoon

Fill a glass with ice, pour in the gin, and top with the ginger ale. Squeeze the juice from the lime wedge and drop it into the drink. Stir gently and serve.

VARIATION: Make the drink into a low-carb Foghorn cocktail by adding an additional ½ ounce of freshly squeezed lime juice. This increases the carbs ever so slightly but adds an extra hint of bitterness.

PER SERVING: CALORIES: 127; TOTAL FAT: 0G; TOTAL CARBOHYDRATES: 0G; FIBER: 0G; PROTEIN: 0G; SUGAR: 0G; SWEETENER CARBS: 0G

# GIN AND TONIC

Although there's no doubt you already know how to whip up a Gin and Tonic, this recipe is here for a good reason. Time after time, keto dieters make the same mistake, assuming tonic water is carb-free, as it looks just like club soda or seltzer. Consider the following a public service announcement for crafting keto cocktails: Regular ol' tonic water is brimming with sugar. Always opt for the diet version.

2 ounces gin

4 ounces diet tonic water, chilled

Lime wedge, for garnish

TOOLS: old-fashioned glass, jigger, bar spoon, paring knife

Fill a glass with ice, pour in the gin, top with the tonic water, and stir well. Squeeze the juice from the lime wedge and drop it into the drink.

VARIATION: If you prefer a sweeter drink, consider using a diet lemon-lime soda instead of tonic water. Other alternatives to the diet tonic water include plain seltzer water, sparkling water, and hard seltzer.

PER SERVING: CALORIES: 127; TOTAL FAT: 0G; TOTAL CARBOHYDRATES: 0G; FIBER: 0G; PROTEIN: 0G; SUGAR: 0G; SWEETENER CARBS: 0G

# BEE'S KNEES

As the name implies, this drink is the absolute best giggle water. The cat's pajamas. The sardine's whiskers. You get the idea! As you might expect, the traditional Bee's Knees is a honey-filled cocktail—full of sugar. To home in on that taste without the carbs, this recipe uses a sugar-free honey-flavor extract. (I like OliveNation brand.)

2 ounces gin

¾ ounce freshly squeezed lemon juice

⅛ teaspoon sugar-free honey flavor extract

Lemon twist, for garnish

TOOLS: shaker, jigger, citrus squeezer, strainer, cocktail glass (chilled), paring knife

Fill a shaker with ice and add the gin, lemon juice, and honey extract. Shake vigorously and strain into a glass. Twist the lemon over the drink, wipe the rim with the lemon, and drop it into the glass.

PREP TIP: Using extracts is a fantastic way to expand the flavors you have on hand, even beyond cocktails. They're so versatile! But if you prefer ready-made, there are sugar-free honey alternatives that actually look and feel like honey. For example, Pyure makes Harmless Hunny, sweetened with stevia.

PER SERVING: CALORIES: 132; TOTAL FAT: 0G; TOTAL CARBOHYDRATES: 1G; FIBER: 0G; PROTEIN: 0G; SUGAR: 1G; SWEETENER CARBS: 0G

# TOM COLLINS

Another classic staple for your growing stockpile of killer cocktail recipes, this popular gin sour is essentially a booze-filled sparkling lemonade. Unlike some of the spin-offs in this book, this recipe stays true to the previously established preparation. The only difference lies in the simple syrup. You'll find premade "Collins mix" at the store, but given the high sugar content, it's best to make your own.

2 ounces gin

1 ounce freshly squeezed lemon juice

½ ounce Low-Carb Simple Syrup (page 116)

3 ounces club soda, chilled

Lemon slice, for garnish

TOOLS: Collins glass, jigger, citrus squeezer, bar spoon

Fill a glass with ice and add the gin, lemon juice, simple syrup, and club soda. Stir gently and garnish with a lemon slice.

VARIATION: Although lemons are traditional in this drink, it can be enjoyed with other citrus fruits, such as lime, grapefruit, and orange.

PER SERVING: CALORIES: 133; TOTAL FAT: 0G; TOTAL CARBOHYDRATES: 2G; FIBER: 0G; PROTEIN: 0G; SUGAR: 1G; SWEETENER CARBS: 8G

# NEGRONI

Ask any bartender or cocktail enthusiast for their top 10 drinks, and the Negroni is sure to make their list. Cliché? Perhaps. Or maybe the drink is just really that damn good. Traditionally made with equal parts gin, Campari, and sweet vermouth, the cocktail clocks more carbs than most keto dieters can reasonably fit within their daily macros. Here, swapping sweet vermouth for dry and ditching the Campari for pomegranate juice keeps the carbs at bay.

2 ounces gin

½ ounce unsweetened pomegranate juice

½ ounce dry vermouth

3 ounces club soda, chilled

Orange twist, for garnish

TOOLS: highball glass, jigger, shaker, strainer, paring knife

Fill a glass with ice. Fill a shaker with ice and add the gin, pomegranate juice, and vermouth. Shake well and strain into the glass. Top with club soda and garnish with an orange twist.

VARIATION: This drink can be made without club soda, or "up" without ice in the glass. If you don't keep vermouth stocked because of its higher carb content, a dry white wine pairs well with the flavors instead. Similarly, if you don't have pomegranate juice on hand, a pomegranate water flavoring will do the trick here.

PER SERVING: CALORIES: 161; TOTAL FAT: 0G; TOTAL CARBOHYDRATES: 4G; FIBER: 0G; PROTEIN: 0G; SUGAR: 3G; SWEETENER CARBS: 0G

# GIMLET

With only two ingredients, gin and Rose's lime juice, this classic cocktail is deceptively unassuming. To make a keto version of Rose's lime juice, pair freshly squeezed lime juice with a low-carb sweetener. Given the minimal ingredients required, this drink is a lifesaver when you're entertaining without a fully stocked bar.

1½ ounces gin

1½ ounces freshly squeezed lime juice

1 teaspoon crystallized allulose or sweetener of choice

Lime wheel, for garnish

**TOOLS:** mixing glass, jigger, citrus squeezer, bar spoon, strainer, cocktail glass (chilled)

Fill a mixing glass with ice and add the gin, lime juice, and sweetener and stir. Strain the drink into a glass and garnish with a lime wheel.

> **VARIATION:** If you have a batch of Low-Carb Simple Syrup (page 116) whipped up, feel free to use ½ ounce of the prepared liquid instead of the solid sweetener. Though gin is the traditional spirit used in this cocktail, a vodka switcheroo will also work wonders.

**PER SERVING:** CALORIES: 108; TOTAL FAT: 0G; TOTAL CARBOHYDRATES: 4G; FIBER: 0G; PROTEIN: 0G; SUGAR: 1G; SWEETENER CARBS: 3G

# BRAMBLE

Since sugary crème de mûre (blackberry liqueur) is not included here, the muddled blackberries infuse the drink with a naturally sweet and earthy flavor instead. For best results, prepare the cocktail in late summer and early fall when fresh blackberries are in season. If fresh blackberries are not an option, thawed frozen berries or berry water flavoring will also do the trick.

8 blackberries

1 ounce freshly squeezed lime juice

1 teaspoon crystallized allulose or sweetener of choice

1½ ounces gin

4 ounces club soda, chilled

Lime wedge, for garnish

---

**TOOLS:** highball glass (chilled), citrus squeezer, muddler, jigger, bar spoon, paring knife

Place the blackberries, lime juice, and sweetener in the bottom of a glass and muddle to combine. Add ice, the gin, and club soda to the glass, then give it a quick stir. Garnish with a lime wedge.

> **VARIATION:** Vodka, white or silver rum, and bourbon are all popular modifications to the traditional gin cocktail. If you want to pack in more of a concentrated berry punch, try adding one or two dashes of blackberry water flavoring, like Stur Blue & Blackberry.

**PER SERVING:** CALORIES: 112; TOTAL FAT: 0G; TOTAL CARBOHYDRATES: 4G; FIBER: 1G; PROTEIN: 0G; SUGAR: 1G; SWEETENER CARBS: 0G

# SINGAPORE SLING

This drink sets the stage for the infamous escapades in the novel and film *Fear and Loathing in Las Vegas*, just before things spiral out of control in "bat country." Rumor has it that the cocktail was author Hunter S. Thompson's drink of choice. All debauchery aside, this is a first-rate classic that belongs in everyone's drink repertoire.

1½ ounces gin

¾ ounce brandy

¾ ounce Low-Carb Orange Liqueur (page 117)

½ ounce freshly squeezed orange juice

½ ounce freshly squeezed lime juice

¼ ounce Bénédictine

3 ounces club soda, chilled

TOOLS: highball glass (chilled), shaker, jigger, citrus squeezer, strainer, bar spoon

Fill a glass with ice. Fill a shaker with ice and add the gin, brandy, orange liqueur, orange juice, lime juice, and Bénédictine. Shake vigorously and strain into the glass. Add the club soda and gently stir.

PREP TIP: This cocktail is traditionally served with a fruity, edible garnish of pineapple, maraschino cherry, and sliced orange. Although the garnish offers a beautiful decorative element, leave it off if you'll be tempted to eat it, as the drink is already a bit high in carbs and may be challenging to align with keto macros.

PER SERVING: CALORIES: 181; TOTAL FAT: 0G; TOTAL CARBOHYDRATES: 3G; FIBER: 0G; PROTEIN: 0G; SUGAR: 1G; SWEETENER CARBS: 4G

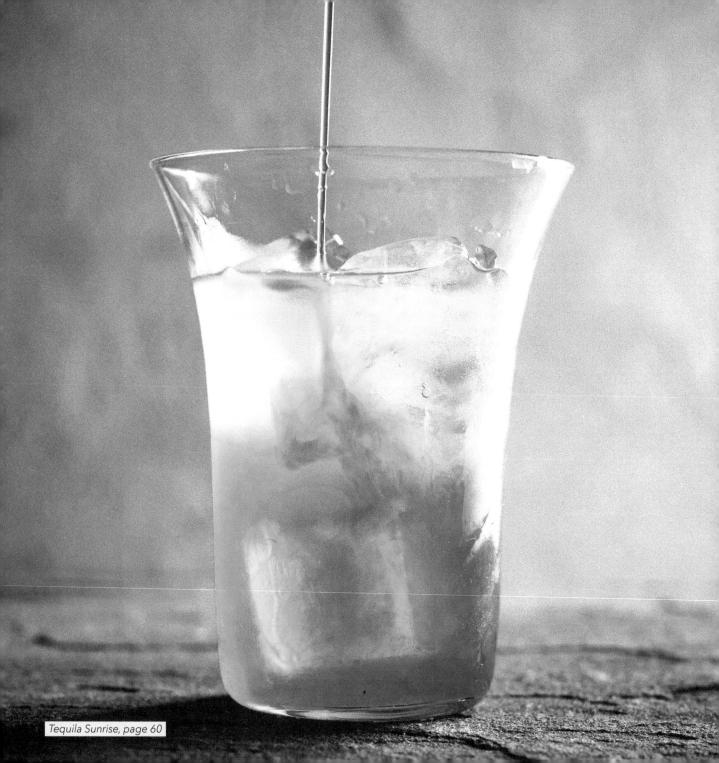

Tequila Sunrise, page 60

# = 6 =
# MEZCAL AND TEQUILA

# TEQUILA SUNRISE

This drink is best known for its iconic sunrise effect, with a colorful transition from red to orange to yellow extending the height of the glass. Traditionally, orange juice serves as the mixer and bright cheery color, while grenadine sweetens the drink and lends the deep red shade to the palette. Keto-friendly replacements include orange sparkling water and unsweetened pomegranate juice.

1½ ounces silver tequila

6 ounces orange-flavored sparkling water

1 teaspoon unsweetened pomegranate juice

2 ounces club soda, chilled (optional)

TOOLS: highball glass, jigger, bar spoon

Fill a glass with ice. Pour in the tequila and sparkling water and stir well. Float the pomegranate juice on top, allowing it to sink into the drink to create a "sunrise" effect. Top with club soda (if using) and serve.

PREP TIP: Another way to create the classic sunrise presentation is to start with the red-colored ingredient on the bottom, in this case pomegranate juice. Then shake the remaining ingredients and strain into the glass.

PER SERVING: CALORIES: 100; TOTAL FAT: 0G; TOTAL CARBOHYDRATES: 1G; FIBER: 0G; PROTEIN: 0G; SUGAR: 1G; SWEETENER CARBS: 0G

# TEQUILA GHOST

If you prefer to sip your tequila cocktails without a brain freeze, give your blender a break and bust out your shaker. Typically made with Pernod, an anise-flavored liqueur, this keto-fied version substitutes a blend of absinthe and low-carb simple syrup to reduce the carb count. The absinthe gives the cocktail an anise-rich flavor and aroma, similar to black licorice.

2 ounces silver tequila

½ ounce absinthe

½ ounce Low-Carb Simple Syrup (page 116)

½ ounce freshly squeezed lemon juice

**TOOLS:** old-fashioned glass, shaker, jigger, citrus squeezer, strainer

Fill a glass with ice. Fill a shaker with ice and add the tequila, absinthe, simple syrup, and lemon juice. Shake vigorously and strain into the glass.

**VARIATION:** Instead of the more costly absinthe, you can achieve similar flavors with more budget-friendly ingredients, such as black licorice flavoring or anise extract. Remember when using extracts that a little goes a long way.

**PER SERVING:** CALORIES: 165; TOTAL FAT: 0G; TOTAL CARBOHYDRATES: 1G; FIBER: 0G; PROTEIN: 0G; SUGAR: 0G; SWEETENER CARBS: 8G

# MATADOR

Traditionally made by shaking an ounce of tequila with two ounces of pineapple juice and a squeeze of lime, this drink is an instant winner. The only problem? Pineapple juice is a sugar bomb. To achieve the pineapple-forward flavors of the classic, use pineapple water flavoring instead of the juice.

½ cup ice

2 ounces gold tequila

½ ounce freshly squeezed lime juice

¼ ounce Low-Carb Simple Syrup, orange variation (page 116)

1½ teaspoons pineapple water flavoring

---

TOOLS: blender, jigger, citrus squeezer, highball glass (chilled)

Add the ice, tequila, lime juice, orange simple syrup, and pineapple flavoring to a blender. Blend until smooth and pour into a glass. Serve immediately.

PREP TIP: You can serve this drink blended or on ice. If you prefer it unblended, add all the ingredients to a shaker and strain into an ice-filled glass.

PER SERVING: CALORIES: 131; TOTAL FAT: 0G; TOTAL CARBOHYDRATES: 1G; FIBER: 0G; PROTEIN: 0G; SUGAR: 0G; SWEETENER CARBS: 4G

# BIRD OF PARADISE

Creamy and sweet, this drink unites almond, vanilla, and chocolate flavors in complete balance. Vanilla extract and unsweetened cacao powder imitate the flavors of customary white crème de cacao, while homemade amaretto does the heavy lifting to replace the high-carb version. This is best served with dessert or enjoyed as a sweet treat on its own.

1½ ounces heavy cream

1 ounce mezcal or tequila

½ ounce Homemade Amaretto (page 119)

¼ teaspoon unsweetened cacao or cocoa powder

⅛ teaspoon vanilla extract

TOOLS: shaker, jigger, strainer, cocktail glass (chilled)

Fill a shaker with ice and add the cream, mezcal, amaretto, cacao powder, and vanilla. Shake well and strain into a glass.

VARIATION: If a batch of homemade amaretto isn't readily available, increase the tequila by ½ ounce, add ⅛ teaspoon of almond extract, and sweeten the cocktail with your preferred sugar substitute.

PER SERVING: CALORIES: 234; TOTAL FAT: 16G; TOTAL CARBOHYDRATES: 1G; FIBER: 0G; PROTEIN: 1G; SUGAR: 1G; SWEETENER CARBS: 6G

# RUDE COSMOPOLITAN

This twist on the classic Cosmopolitan (page 88) swaps out the vodka for tequila. With its light pink color, it may look a little tame, but beware. It's a remarkably stiff drink, so sip with caution! The classic version uses cranberry juice and triple sec or Cointreau. This adaptation uses diet cranberry juice and homemade low-carb orange liqueur to keep the carbs in check.

2 ounces gold tequila

1½ ounces diet cranberry juice

1 ounce Low-Carb Orange Liqueur (page 117)

½ ounce freshly squeezed lime juice

TOOLS: shaker, jigger, citrus squeezer, strainer, cocktail glass (chilled)

Fill a shaker with ice and add the tequila, cranberry juice, orange liqueur, and lime juice. Shake well and strain into a glass.

> VARIATION: The orange liqueur can be swapped out for the orange variation of Low-Carb Simple Syrup (page 116) if preferred. Either is outstanding!

PER SERVING: CALORIES: 200; TOTAL FAT: 0G; TOTAL CARBOHYDRATES: 6G; FIBER: 0G; PROTEIN: 0G; SUGAR: 5G; SWEETENER CARBS: 5G

# HOT PANTS

Incredibly short shorts or most underrated cocktail of all time? You decide. Balancing tequila with grapefruit and peppermint in perfect harmony, this cocktail successfully marries outwardly opposing flavors. It's an unexpected marriage to be sure, but it works so well. Traditionally made with peppermint schnapps and powdered sugar, the keto version uses peppermint tea and allulose.

Lemon wedge, for garnish

Kosher salt, for garnish

2 ounces tequila or mezcal

1 ounce unsweetened brewed peppermint tea, chilled

¾ ounce fresh grapefruit juice

1 teaspoon powdered allulose or sweetener of choice

TOOLS: old-fashioned glass (chilled), shaker, jigger, strainer

Moisten the rim of a glass with the lime. Dip the rim into the salt and set aside. Fill a shaker with ice and add the tequila, peppermint tea, grapefruit juice, and allulose. Shake well and strain into the glass.

VARIATION: Grapefruit water flavoring can replace fresh grapefruit juice if preferred, which will lower the carbs even further. Peppermint tea can be substituted with ⅛ teaspoon of peppermint extract if needed.

PER SERVING: CALORIES: 135; TOTAL FAT: 0G; TOTAL CARBOHYDRATES: 2G; FIBER: 0G; PROTEIN: 0G; SUGAR: 2G; SWEETENER CARBS: 4G

# AVOCADO MARGARITA

The buttery flavor of avocado softens the nip of tequila while adding a rich, creamy texture to the cocktail that's oh so luxurious. Besides, avocado is a nutritional powerhouse, so you're loading up on vitamins, minerals, and healthy fats with each sip. Think of it as a boozy keto smoothie. The low-carb Margarita Mix (page 121) is a great shortcut for entertaining a thirsty crowd.

½ cup ice

¼ cup diced avocado

1½ ounces silver tequila

1 ounce heavy cream

½ ounce Low-Carb Orange Liqueur (page 117)

½ ounce freshly squeezed lime juice

TOOLS: blender, paring knife, jigger, citrus squeezer, cocktail glass (chilled)

Add the ice, avocado, tequila, cream, orange liqueur, and lime juice to a blender. Blend until smooth and pour into a glass. Serve immediately.

VARIATION: To accommodate dairy-free dietary restrictions, swap out the cream for unsweetened coconut cream or milk. And if you don't have a batch of Low-Carb Orange Liqueur at the ready, Low-Carb Simple Syrup (page 116) or any keto sweetener will be fantastic.

PER SERVING: CALORIES: 283; TOTAL FAT: 16G; TOTAL CARBOHYDRATES: 5G; FIBER: 3G; PROTEIN: 1G; SUGAR: 1G; SWEETENER CARBS: 3G

# EL DIABLO

*El diablo* means "the devil" in Spanish, though the cocktail isn't nearly as foreboding as its name. For something that sounds like it will hit your taste buds with a fiery blow, the drink is ironically mellow and fairly sweet. An El Diablo actually earns its title from the dark red crème de cassis liqueur typically used to make it. We use pomegranate juice in place of cassis to achieve the distinctive red coloring without racking up carbs.

1½ ounces mezcal
  or tequila

½ ounce freshly squeezed
  lime juice

½ ounce Low-Carb Simple
  Syrup (page 116)

½ ounce unsweetened
  pomegranate juice

4 ounces diet ginger
  ale, chilled

**TOOLS:** old-fashioned
glass, jigger, citrus
squeezer, bar spoon

Fill a glass with ice and add the mezcal, lime juice, simple syrup, and pomegranate juice. Top with ginger ale and gently stir.

> **VARIATION:** Berry or pomegranate water flavoring or extracts may be used to replace the pomegranate juice. Only a small amount of either is necessary; start with a dash and work up to achieve the desired flavor.

**PER SERVING:** CALORIES: 108; TOTAL FAT: 0.5G; TOTAL CARBOHYDRATES: 3G; FIBER: 0G; PROTEIN: 0G; SUGAR: 2G; SWEETENER CARBS: 8G

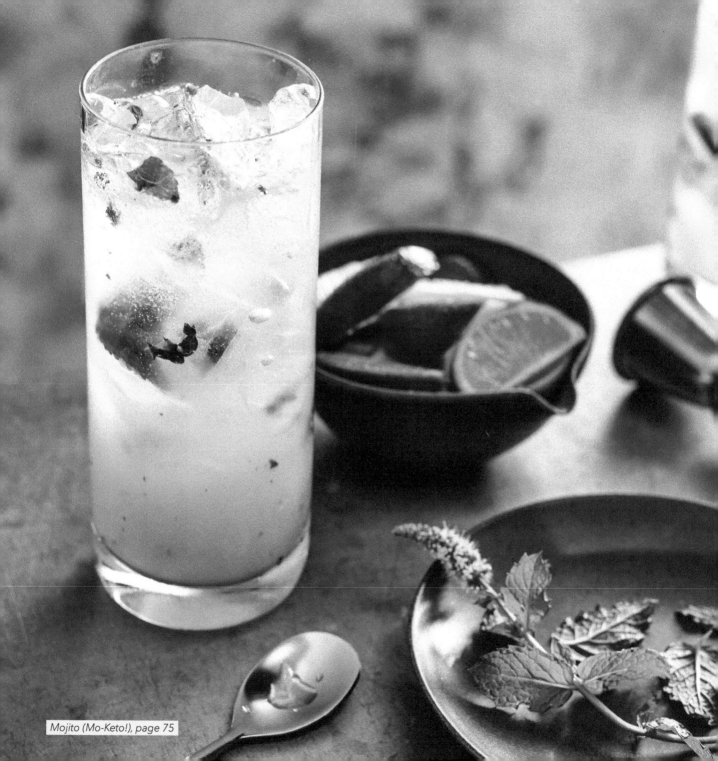

Mojito (Mo-Keto!), page 75

# = 7 =
# RUM

# HOT BUTTERED RUM

**MAKES 4 DRINKS**

Unlike most rum drinks you'll come across, this one is not frosty, fruity, or tropical, but warm and heavy—something to grab a book and cozy up with. In classic form, brown sugar or honey sweeten the cocktail, but all the other ingredients are good to go for keto. You'll get all the traditional flavors of the original while minimizing carbs with a simple sweetener swap.

2 cups water

4 tablespoons (½ stick) unsalted butter

¼ cup monk fruit blend with erythritol or sweetener of choice

1 teaspoon ground cinnamon

½ teaspoon ground nutmeg

½ teaspoon sea salt

1 cup dark rum

**TOOLS:** large saucepan, Irish coffee mug, whisk

Combine the water, butter, sweetener, cinnamon, nutmeg, and salt in a large saucepan over medium-high heat. Bring to a boil, then reduce the heat and simmer over low heat, whisking well, for 5 minutes. Remove from the heat, carefully pour in the rum, and stir well. Serve in mugs or heatproof glassware while still warm.

> **VARIATION:** Although this is the classic that we all know and love, consider switching spirits for a unique spin that will knock your fuzzy socks off. Hot Buttered Brandy? Hot Buttered Whiskey? Yes, please!

**PER SERVING:** CALORIES: 363; TOTAL FAT: 12G; TOTAL CARBOHYDRATES: 1G; FIBER: 0G; PROTEIN: 0G; SUGAR: 0G; SWEETENER CARBS: 12G

# THE TEMPEST

This Dark and Stormy spin-off is essentially a Caribbean riff on the Moscow Mule (page 84), using dark rum instead of vodka. Traditionally, the drink mixes Gosling's Black Seal Rum from Bermuda with ginger beer and simple syrup. Any dark rum will do the trick with this recipe, though you'll need diet ginger beer and low-carb simple syrup to build this drink. The preparation is straight-forward, making this cocktail ideal for easy entertaining.

2 ounces dark rum

½ ounce Low-Carb Simple Syrup (page 116)

4 ounces diet ginger beer

Lime wedge

TOOLS: old-fashioned glass, jigger, bar spoon, paring knife

Fill a glass with ice. Add the rum and simple syrup to the glass and stir well. Top with ginger beer. Squeeze the juice from the lime wedge into the glass and drop it into the drink.

VARIATION: Knock the ginger flavor and aroma up a few levels by adding slices of fresh ginger to the drink. Just slip the ginger in with the ice before adding the liquid ingredients.

PER SERVING: CALORIES: 127; TOTAL FAT: 0G; TOTAL CARBOHYDRATES: 0G; FIBER: 0G; PROTEIN: 0G; SUGAR: 0G; SWEETENER CARBS: 8G

# PIÑA COLADA

The name Piña Colada, which translates to "strained pineapple" in Spanish, is a reference to the fresh pineapple juice traditionally used in the cocktail. However, using coconut-pineapple-flavored sparkling water significantly cuts back the sugar while giving the coconut flavor a boost. Swapping in canned coconut milk for the sweetened coconut cream also helps reduce carbs. This fruity cocktail is a tropical classic to enjoy poolside, while sunbathing, or whenever the earworm-y song blasts through your speakers.

6 ounces coconut-pineapple-flavored sparkling water

½ cup ice

2 ounces light rum

2 ounces canned full-fat coconut milk

½ ounce Low-Carb Simple Syrup (page 116)

TOOLS: blender, jigger, hurricane or highball glass, cocktail umbrella (optional), wide straw (optional)

Add the sparkling water, ice, rum, coconut milk, and simple syrup to a blender. Blend until smooth and pour into a glass. Serve with a cocktail umbrella (if using) and a wide straw (if using) and go get caught in the rain.

> PREP TIP: Though the blended piña colada probably first comes to mind when you think of this cocktail, the drink is commonly prepared shaken. Add all the ingredients to an ice-filled shaker, shake-shake-shake, then strain into a chilled glass.

PER SERVING: CALORIES: 239; TOTAL FAT: 12G; TOTAL CARBOHYDRATES: 2G; FIBER: 0G; PROTEIN: 1G; SUGAR: 0G; SWEETENER CARBS: 8G

# ACAPULCO

This cocktail delivers a fresh spin on warm-weather rum drinks. The combination of light rum, frothy egg white, lime, and mint produces a cool and refreshing tonic to enjoy while you play in the sun or relax in the shade. Cointreau and simple syrup are typically used to build the drink, but low-carb orange liqueur serves as an incredible substitute for both in this adaptation.

1½ ounces light rum

1 large egg white

½ ounce Low-Carb Orange Liqueur (page 117)

½ ounce freshly squeezed lime juice

Mint sprig, for garnish

TOOLS: shaker, jigger, citrus squeezer, strainer, cocktail glass (chilled)

Combine the rum, egg white, orange liqueur, and lime juice in a shaker. Shake vigorously for at least 30 seconds. Add ice and shake a second time. Strain into a glass and garnish with a mint sprig.

> VARIATION: If using raw egg whites is out of your comfort zone, consider opting for powdered egg whites instead to achieve the same airy, whipped consistency. Or omit the egg whites altogether—the cocktail is still tasty without the frothy texture.

PER SERVING: CALORIES: 142; TOTAL FAT: 0G; TOTAL CARBOHYDRATES: 1G; FIBER: 0G; PROTEIN: 4G; SUGAR: 0G; SWEETENER CARBS: 3G

# BAHAMA MAMA

This tropical drink is fruity and fun, making it perfect for parties and warm weather gatherings. It's also great for pretending you're on an exotic vacation while you sip away in your living room! To reduce the sugar content of the drink, coconut-pineapple-flavored sparkling water replaces both pineapple juice and the coconut rum typically used. Low-carb coffee liqueur is put to work in place of regular coffee liqueur to keep carbs down.

5 ounces coconut-pineapple-flavored sparkling water

2 ounces dark rum

1 ounce freshly squeezed lemon juice

½ ounce Low-Carb Coffee Liqueur (page 118)

Pineapple leaf, for garnish

Lemon slice, for garnish

TOOLS: shaker, jigger, citrus squeezer, strainer, hurricane or highball glass (chilled)

Fill a shaker with ice and add the sparkling water, rum, lemon juice, and coffee liqueur. Shake the ingredients vigorously and strain into a glass. Garnish with a pineapple leaf and a slice of lemon.

> PREP TIP: Ditch the shaker and bust out the blender; this cocktail is a fantastic blended drink. Blend ½ cup of ice with the sparkling water, rum, lemon juice, and coffee liqueur and pour into a chilled glass.

PER SERVING: CALORIES: 145; TOTAL FAT: 0G; TOTAL CARBOHYDRATES: 2G; FIBER: 0G; PROTEIN: 0G; SUGAR: 1G: SWEETENER CARBS: 5G

# MOJITO (MO-KETO!)

With all the cocktail recipes in this book, you'd think it would be hard for me to pick a favorite. But this spin on the classic recipe has served me well over the years. Inspired by a local happy hour special, I set out to create a keto version years ago and have since tweaked it to perfection. It's my top cocktail of choice, hands down. The original version is posted on my website (and made with vodka!) if you're interested in seeing how the recipe has evolved.

8 mint leaves, plus 1 mint sprig, for garnish

1 ounce freshly squeezed lime juice

1 tablespoon crystallized allulose or sweetener of choice

2 ounces light rum

4 ounces club soda, chilled

**TOOLS:** highball glass, citrus squeezer, muddler, jigger

Place the mint leaves in the bottom of a glass. Add the lime juice and sweetener and muddle well to crush the leaves and dissolve the sweetener. Add the rum to the glass and fill it with ice. Top with club soda and garnish with a sprig of mint to serve.

PREP TIP: The type of mint leaves used has a subtle influence on the cocktail's aroma and flavor. There are a variety of mints readily available at the grocery store or farmers' market to experiment with: spearmint, peppermint, lemon balm, apple mint, and ginger mint, to name just a few.

PER SERVING: CALORIES: 135; TOTAL FAT: 0G; TOTAL CARBOHYDRATES: 2G; FIBER: 0G; PROTEIN: 0G; SUGAR: 0G: SWEETENER CARBS: 12G

# CAIPIRISSIMA

Slightly sweet with a burst of fresh citrus, this cocktail is reminiscent of lime-ade with a boozy bite. The keto rendition remains faithful to the classic (not counting allulose replacing turbinado sugar). Naturally, you can enjoy this drink year-round, but sipping under the stars in the warm summer breeze is preferable.

½ lime, cut into 4 wedges

2 teaspoons crystallized allulose or sweetener of choice

2 ounces rum

TOOLS: paring knife, old-fashioned glass, muddler, jigger, bar spoon

Place the lime wedges at the bottom of a glass and sprinkle the allulose over the top. Mash the ingredients with a muddler to dissolve the sweetener and release the lime juice. Fill the glass with ice, leaving the muddled fruit at the bottom. Pour in the rum and give the drink a quick stir.

VARIATION: When muddling is involved, there's always an opportunity for creative adjustments. Consider combining the lime wedges with lemon or tossing in a few berries for a Bramble-esque (page 55) twist.

PER SERVING: CALORIES: 133; TOTAL FAT: 0G; TOTAL CARBOHYDRATES: 2G; FIBER: 0G; PROTEIN: 0G; SUGAR: 0G; SWEETENER CARBS: 8G

# STRAWBERRY DAIQUIRI

If you're a fan of smoothies, you will love this daiquiri recipe. A classic daiquiri combines rum, lime juice, and simple syrup. The addition of frozen strawberries and strawberry water flavoring keeps carbs minimal while packing in as much strawberry flavor as possible. And naturally, our trusty low-carb simple syrup sweetens everything up.

¼ cup frozen whole strawberries

¼ cup ice

2 ounces light rum

½ ounce freshly squeezed lime juice

½ ounce Low-Carb Simple Syrup (page 116)

½ teaspoon strawberry water flavoring (optional)

TOOLS: blender, jigger, citrus squeezer, cocktail glass (chilled)

Add the strawberries, ice, rum, lime juice, simple syrup, and strawberry flavoring (if using) to a blender. Blend until smooth and pour into a glass. Serve immediately.

> VARIATION: For a more traditional daiquiri flavor, skip the water flavoring and swap out the frozen strawberries for more ice (a total of ½ cup).

PER SERVING: CALORIES: 155; TOTAL FAT: 0G; TOTAL CARBOHYDRATES: 6G; FIBER: 1G; PROTEIN: 0G; SUGAR: 3G; SWEETENER CARBS: 8G

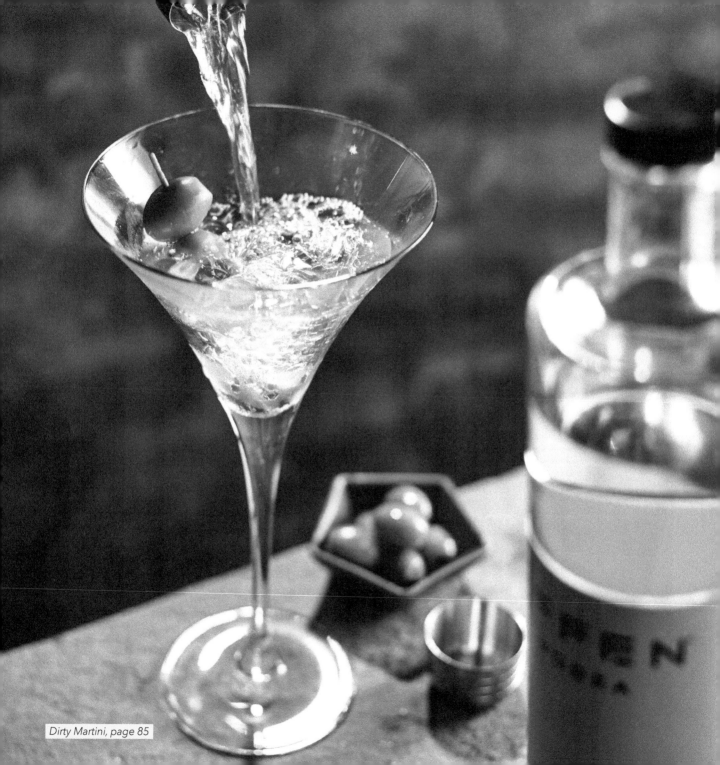

*Dirty Martini, page 85*

# = 8 =
# VODKA

# EASY BREEZY

This is a mishmash of a traditional Bay Breeze (rum, cranberry juice, and pineapple juice) and a Sea Breeze (vodka, cranberry juice, and grapefruit juice). Instead of the usual high-sugar ingredients, diet cranberry juice, pineapple water flavoring, and coconut-pineapple-flavored sparkling water are mixed with vodka to give this drink a unique spin.

1½ ounces vodka

1 ounce diet
   cranberry juice

½ teaspoon pineapple
   water flavoring

4 ounces
   coconut-pineapple-
   flavored sparkling water

TOOLS: highball glass,
jigger, bar spoon

Fill a glass with ice and add the vodka, cranberry juice, pineapple flavoring, and sparkling water. Stir well.

VARIATION: Try flipping the ratio of the ingredients, mixing 4 ounces of diet cranberry juice with 1 ounce of coconut-pineapple-flavored sparkling water. The resulting drink will be a pleasantly tart version of the Easy Breezy. You can also make a more classic rendition of a Bay Breeze by swapping the vodka for light rum.

PER SERVING: CALORIES: 97; TOTAL FAT: 0G; TOTAL CARBOHYDRATES: 0G; FIBER: 0G; PROTEIN: 0G; SUGAR: 0G; SWEETENER CARBS: 0G

# WHITE SPIDER

A vodka stinger cocktail such as this usually uses only two ingredients: a mint-based liqueur and a spirit. The liqueur is often crème de menthe or peppermint schnapps, though the spirit varies. The traditional liqueurs are too sugary, but a mix of low-carb simple syrup and peppermint extract can serve as an excellent replacement. Instead of the extract, you can also use chilled peppermint tea or muddled fresh peppermint leaves.

2 ounces vodka

1 ounce Low-Carb Simple Syrup (page 116)

⅛ teaspoon peppermint extract

Peppermint sprig, for garnish

TOOLS: shaker, jigger, strainer, cocktail glass (chilled)

Fill a shaker with ice and add the vodka, simple syrup, and peppermint extract. Shake vigorously and strain into a glass. Garnish with a sprig of fresh peppermint laid on top.

PREP TIP: To make the drink less potent, serve on the rocks in a Collins or highball glass and top with diet tonic water.

PER SERVING: CALORIES: 129; TOTAL FAT: 0G; TOTAL CARBOHYDRATES: 0G; FIBER: 0G; PROTEIN: 0G; SUGAR: 0G; SWEETENER CARBS: 16G

# WHITE RUSSIAN

If you've seen the cult-classic film *The Big Lebowski*, then it should come as no surprise that this is The Dude's favorite drink. He's seen mixing and sipping a White Russian or sporting a frothy white mustache in nearly every scene of the movie, typically while dropping some very quotable lines. But you don't need to have seen the movie to love this drink!

2 ounces vodka

1 ounce Low-Carb Coffee Liqueur (page 118)

1 ounce heavy cream

TOOLS: old-fashioned glass, jigger, bar spoon

Fill a glass with ice. Pour in the vodka and coffee liqueur and stir well. Float the cream on the top and serve. The Dude abides.

VARIATION: To make a Black Russian, skip the cream. Instead, shake the vodka and coffee liqueur with ice, strain into an ice-filled glass, and finish with a lemon twist.

PER SERVING: CALORIES: 251; TOTAL FAT: 11G; TOTAL CARBOHYDRATES: 1G; FIBER: 0G; PROTEIN: 1G; SUGAR: 1G; SWEETENER CARBS: 9G

# MUDSLIDE

Kahlúa and Baileys Irish Cream are standard components of the drink, but homemade low-carb coffee liqueur serves as a marvelous substitute in this adaptation. This can be enjoyed as a frozen blended drink (as this is) or served on the rocks after a firm shaking. The former is essentially a boozy milkshake, whereas the latter is more similar to a White Russian (page 82).

½ cup ice

1½ ounces Low-Carb Coffee Liqueur (page 118)

1 ounce vodka

1 ounce heavy cream

½ ounce whiskey

½ teaspoon unsweetened cocoa powder

**TOOLS:** blender, jigger, wine glass (chilled)

Add the ice, coffee liqueur, vodka, cream, whiskey, and cocoa powder to a blender. Blend until smooth. Pour into a glass and serve immediately.

> **MAKE IT A MOCKTAIL:** Skip the booze and turn your Mudslide into a DIY blended coffee instead: ½ cup ice, 2 ounces cold brew coffee, 2 ounces heavy cream, ½ ounce Low-Carb Simple Syrup (page 116), and ½ teaspoon unsweetened cocoa powder. And by all means, increase the coffee if you need a caffeine boost.

**PER SERVING:** CALORIES: 228; TOTAL FAT: 11G; TOTAL CARBOHYDRATES: 1G; FIBER: 0G; PROTEIN: 1G; SUGAR: 1G; SWEETENER CARBS: 13G

# MOSCOW MULE

This cocktail is outstanding—if not for its crisp, effervescent consistency and zingy flavor, then for the utter simplicity of its preparation. Ultra-casual and full of pep, a Moscow Mule is the perfect refreshment to liven up any relaxed get-together. Instead of ginger beer, diet ginger beer or diet ginger ale is used to lower the carb count. Serving the cocktail in a copper mug is traditional and adds to the visual presentation of the drink, but any glassware will suffice.

2 ounces Russian vodka

½ ounce freshly squeezed lime juice

4 ounces diet ginger beer or diet ginger ale

TOOLS: copper mug or highball glass, jigger, citrus squeezer, bar spoon

Fill a mug with ice and pour in the vodka and lime juice. Top with ginger beer and stir.

VARIATION: Just as "Moscow" is a clue that there is Russian vodka in this cocktail, variations using other spirits have names that reflect their associated locales—a Mexican Mule uses tequila, and bourbon makes a Kentucky Mule.

PER SERVING: CALORIES: 129; TOTAL FAT: 0G; TOTAL CARBOHYDRATES: 1G; FIBER: 0G; PROTEIN: 0G; SUGAR: 0G; SWEETENER CARBS: 0G

# DIRTY MARTINI

No keto adaptations are necessary for this classic! The traditional recipe is low enough in carbs that you can enjoy it as is. Dry vermouth is the ingredient with the highest carb count, but it's used in such a minuscule quantity that it has almost no impact on the total carbs. This is an outstanding example of how to offset the sugar in higher-carb ingredients by reducing their volume and opting for more keto-friendly choices.

2 ounces vodka

½ ounce dry vermouth

½ ounce green olive brine

3 green olives

TOOLS: shaker, jigger, strainer, cocktail glass (chilled), cocktail skewer

Fill a shaker with ice and add the vodka, vermouth, and olive brine. Shake vigorously and strain into a glass. Thread the green olives onto a cocktail skewer and drop into the glass.

PREP TIP: Martinis can be shaken or stirred, though many people have a preference for one or the other. If you prefer stirring over shaking, switch the shaker for a mixing glass and bar spoon, stir all the ingredients together, and strain into the cocktail glass.

PER SERVING: CALORIES: 163; TOTAL FAT: 1G; TOTAL CARBOHYDRATES: 2G; FIBER: 0G; PROTEIN: 0G; SUGAR: 0G; SWEETENER CARBS: 0G

# CAPE CODDER

The Cape Codder, or Cape Cod, is one of the most popular drinks of our time. Often referred to as a "vodka cranberry," the drink is exactly that: vodka and cranberry juice. Occasionally lime and club soda are mixed in, but it's the winning flavor combination of cranberry with vodka that makes the drink a mainstay in bars around the world. The low-carb rendition of the cocktail uses diet cranberry juice to keep all the cranberry flavor without the carbs.

5 ounces diet cranberry juice

2 ounces vodka

½ ounce freshly squeezed lime juice

½ ounce club soda, chilled (optional)

**TOOLS:** highball glass, jigger, citrus squeezer, shaker, strainer

Fill a glass with ice. Fill a shaker with ice and add the cranberry juice, vodka, and lime juice. Shake well and strain into the glass. Finish with a splash of club soda (if using) to add a hint of carbonation.

**PREP TIP:** If you prefer, you can skip the shaker and mix this drink directly in the highball glass. Fill the glass with ice, add the liquids, and stir gently.

**PER SERVING:** CALORIES: 133; TOTAL FAT: 0G; TOTAL CARBOHYDRATES: 1G; FIBER: 0G; PROTEIN: 0G; SUGAR: 0G; SWEETENER CARBS: 0G

# PINK LEMONADE

Sipping a spiked pink lemonade is a brilliant way to unwind on a sweltering summer day. Although most lemonades are filled with plenty of sugar, the carbs are minimal in this warm-weather cocktail thanks to low-carb simple syrup, diet juice, and diet soda. If you prefer your lemonade to be more tart than sweet, consider using club soda in place of the diet soda.

1½ ounces vodka

1 ounce diet cranberry juice

1 ounce freshly squeezed lemon juice

½ ounce Low-Carb Simple Syrup, orange variation (page 116)

5 ounces diet lemon-lime soda, chilled

TOOLS: Collins glass, shaker, jigger, citrus squeezer, strainer, bar spoon

Fill a glass with ice. Fill a shaker with ice and add the vodka, cranberry juice, lemon juice, and orange simple syrup. Shake well and strain into the glass. Top with the lemon-lime soda and gently stir.

MAKE IT A MOCKTAIL: For a refreshing nonalcoholic beverage, just omit the vodka.

PER SERVING: CALORIES: 104; TOTAL FAT: 0G; TOTAL CARBOHYDRATES: 2G; FIBER: 0G; PROTEIN: 0G; SUGAR: 1G; SWEETENER CARBS: 8G

# COSMOPOLITAN

Commonly referred to merely as a "Cosmo," this popular modern cocktail has become permanently cemented in pop-culture canon thanks to the hit TV series *Sex and the City*. With its pretty pink hue and ease going down, it's no surprise this was everyone's drink of choice on the show. The original is made with Cointreau, lime, and cranberry juice, but the keto rendition makes use of low-carb orange liqueur, diet cranberry juice, and fresh citrus. Any old vodka will work well, but citron vodka is a popular choice for this beverage.

1½ ounces vodka

1½ ounces Low-Carb Orange Liqueur (page 117)

½ ounce freshly squeezed lime juice

½ ounce freshly squeezed lemon juice

2 dashes diet cranberry juice

Lemon twist, for garnish

TOOLS: shaker, jigger, citrus squeezer, strainer, cocktail glass (chilled), paring knife

Fill a shaker with ice and add the vodka, orange liqueur, lime juice, lemon juice, and cranberry juice. Shake well and strain into a glass. Twist the lemon over the drink, wipe the rim with the lemon, and drop it into the glass.

VARIATION: Popular variations of the Cosmopolitan highlight the cranberry juice, amping up the volume of cranberry flavoring while pulling back on other flavors. For a Cranberry Cosmo, use 1 ounce of diet cranberry juice and halve the citrus-based ingredients. For a Crantini, make the Cranberry Cosmo and add an extra ounce of diet cranberry juice.

PER SERVING: CALORIES: 174; TOTAL FAT: 0G; TOTAL CARBOHYDRATES: 2G; FIBER: 0G; PROTEIN: 0G; SUGAR: 1G; SWEETENER CARBS: 7G

# LEMON DROP

This cocktail is tart and sweet, with a flavor profile strikingly similar to the popular lemony hard candies of the same name. The drink's sweetness lends itself to a dessert pairing, but it can be enjoyed on any occasion. Typically made with Grand Marnier or Cointreau, sugar, and orange juice, the classic is reinterpreted here with low-carb orange liqueur and allulose to reduce the carbs.

Crystallized allulose or sweetener of choice, for garnish

Lemon wedge, for garnish

1½ ounces vodka

1 ounce Low-Carb Orange Liqueur (page 117)

1 ounce freshly squeezed lemon juice

**TOOLS:** small plate, paring knife, cocktail glass (chilled), shaker, jigger, citrus squeezer, strainer

Pour a layer of allulose on a small plate. Moisten the rim of a glass with a lemon wedge (reserve for garnish), dip the rim into the allulose, and set aside. Fill a shaker with ice and add the vodka, orange liqueur, and lemon juice. Shake well and strain into the glass. Float the lemon wedge in the drink to garnish.

> **VARIATION:** For an on-the-rocks version of this cocktail, trade out the cocktail glass for an ice-filled highball glass and top with chilled club soda or lemon sparkling water.

**PER SERVING:** CALORIES: 150; TOTAL FAT: 0G; TOTAL CARBOHYDRATES: 2G; FIBER: 0G; PROTEIN: 0G; SUGAR: 1G; SWEETENER CARBS: 5G

# BLOODY MARY

This is traditionally served as a breakfast cocktail, equal parts hair of the dog and nutrient-boosting meal. Although the drink's ability to cure hangovers is questionable, the cocktail is undeniably satisfying. Many variations exist, but vodka and tomato juice are staple ingredients for them all. If you're mixing up multiple Bloody Marys, save yourself some time and carbs by whipping up a large batch of the keto Bloody Mary mix.

Salt, for garnish (optional)

Lemon wedge, for garnish

4 ounces Bloody Mary Mix (page 120)

2 ounces vodka or bacon-infused vodka

3 green olives, for garnish

1 celery stalk, for garnish

1 bacon slice, cooked, for garnish

TOOLS: small plate, paring knife, highball glass, shaker, jigger, strainer, cocktail skewer

Pour a layer of salt on a small plate. Moisten the rim of the glass with the lemon wedge (reserve for garnish) and dip the rim into the salt. Fill the glass with ice. Fill a shaker with ice and add the Bloody Mary Mix and vodka, then shake well. Strain into the glass. Thread the olives onto a cocktail skewer and garnish with the lemon wedge, celery stalk, and bacon slice.

PREP TIP: Unlike many garnishes, Bloody Mary trimmings are more than ornamental, they are often full-blown meals. It's not uncommon to see these cocktails sporting keto-friendly snacks on top, like grilled kebabs, pickled veggies, peppers, chicken wings, meatballs, ribs, or deviled eggs. Let your culinary creativity run wild and swap out the garnishes as you see fit.

PER SERVING: CALORIES: 210; TOTAL FAT: 5G; TOTAL CARBOHYDRATES: 4G; FIBER: 2G; PROTEIN: 4G; SUGAR: 2G; SWEETENER CARBS: 0G

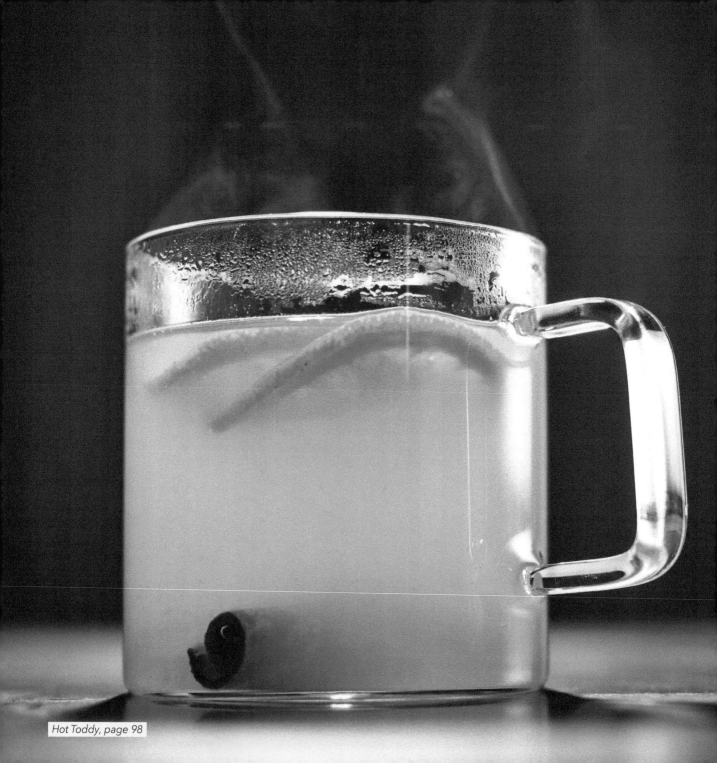

*Hot Toddy, page 98*

# = 9 =
# WHISKEY

# WHISKEY HIGHBALL

A highball cocktail is known to have only two basic ingredients, a spirit and a carbonated mixer, served over ice in a tall glass. Popular highball drinks include rum and coke, seven and seven, and Gin and Tonic (page 50). A whiskey highball follows suit, where the whiskey is typically combined with ginger ale, though you can use other carbonated drinks. Any kind of whiskey will work well with this simple drink, so you are welcome to choose whatever you prefer.

1½ ounces whiskey

5 ounces diet ginger ale

Lemon twist, for garnish (optional)

TOOLS: highball glass, jigger, bar spoon

Fill a glass with ice and pour in the whiskey. Top with ginger ale and stir gently. Twist the lemon (if using) over the drink, wipe the rim with the lemon, and drop it into the glass.

VARIATION: Not a fan of ginger? Replace the ginger ale with your carbonated beverage of choice—seltzer, club soda, and diet sodas are all great options. If you choose a mixer that lacks sweetness, consider adding some Low-Carb Simple Syrup (page 116) to balance the drink.

PER SERVING: CALORIES: 97; TOTAL FAT: 0G; TOTAL CARBOHYDRATES: 0G; FIBER: 0G; PROTEIN: 0G; SUGAR: 0G; SWEETENER CARBS: 0G

# MINT JULEP

The "right" way to make a mint julep is hotly debated, but I'd argue that you can't go wrong with any of them! Whether opting for a simple glass of bourbon with a single sprig of mint, muddling several sprigs of spearmint to oblivion, infusing bourbon directly with mint, or combining everything in a blender, it's all A-OK. There are two crucial things you'll need regardless of which style you choose: Kentucky bourbon and fresh mint.

14 mint leaves, plus 2 mint sprigs, for garnish

1 ounce Low-Carb Simple Syrup (page 116)

4 ounces Kentucky bourbon

TOOLS: julep cup or old-fashioned glass, muddler, jigger, bar spoon

Place the mint leaves and simple syrup in a glass and muddle them together. Add crushed ice and pour in the bourbon. Stir well, until the glass frosts. Slip the mint sprigs into the drink to garnish and serve.

VARIATION: Make a mint julep slushie by blending the drink with 1 ounce of freshly squeezed lemon juice and ½ cup of ice. Muddle the mint, sweetener, and bourbon, then place in a blender. Add the lemon juice and ice, blend until smooth, and pour into a chilled glass to serve.

PER SERVING: CALORIES: 258; TOTAL FAT: 0G; TOTAL CARBOHYDRATES: 0G; FIBER: 0G; PROTEIN: 0G; SUGAR: 0G; SWEETENER CARBS: 16G

# OLD-FASHIONED

This cocktail is a timeless classic, made with muddled citrus, sugar, and bitters to balance the whiskey. It is customary to use bourbon as the spirit, though blended whiskey, Scotch, and rye work well, too. The traditional sugar is swapped for allulose (or use your preferred low-carb sweetener). Be sure to very thinly cut the orange slice to limit the carbs.

½ very thin orange slice

1 teaspoon crystallized allulose or sweetener of choice

1 teaspoon water

3 dashes Angostura bitters

2½ ounces bourbon

Orange twist, for garnish

**TOOLS:** old-fashioned glass, muddler, jigger, bar spoon, paring knife

Place the orange slice, allulose, water, and bitters in the bottom of a glass and muddle together. Fill the glass with ice, pour in the bourbon, and stir. Swipe the rim with the orange peel, twist to release the oils over the drink, and garnish.

> **VARIATION:** For a more "old-fashioned" Old-Fashioned, use lemon instead of orange. Switch out the orange slice for lemon zest and finish the drink with a lemon twist.

**PER SERVING:** CALORIES: 161; TOTAL FAT: 0G; TOTAL CARBOHYDRATES: 0G; FIBER: 0G; PROTEIN: 0G; SUGAR: 0G; SWEETENER CARBS: 4G

# SAZERAC

A Sazerac was originally prepared with a simple combination of Cognac and Peychaud's bitters. Over the years, the cocktail has evolved into a more elaborate mix of ingredients, including sugar cubes, absinthe (or Pernod or Herbsaint), fresh citrus, and occasionally bourbon as the star spirit. The keto rendition swaps out the sugar cubes for allulose and opts for absinthe instead of Pernod or Herbsaint, both relatively high in carbs. On the other hand, if you don't have absinthe, you may use either liqueur, as the 1 teaspoon used in the drink has no real impact.

1 teaspoon crystallized allulose or sweetener of choice

2 dashes Peychaud's or Angostura bitters

2 ounces bourbon or Cognac

½ ounce freshly squeezed lemon juice

1 teaspoon absinthe or Pernod (see Variation, page 61)

Lemon twist, for garnish

TOOLS: old-fashioned glass, jigger, citrus squeezer, bar spoon, paring knife

Saturate the allulose with the bitters in a glass. Fill the glass with ice and add the bourbon, lemon juice, and absinthe and stir. Swipe the rim with the lemon peel, twist to release the oils over the drink, and garnish.

VARIATION: This recipe is in line with a New Orleans-style version of the Sazerac. For a more classic rendition, scrap the sweetener and lemon juice. Pour a little absinthe or Pernod into a glass and swirl it to coat the glass, then dump the excess. Shake the bourbon with ice and a few dashes of bitters, then strain into the coated glass.

PER SERVING: CALORIES: 132; TOTAL FAT: 0G; TOTAL CARBOHYDRATES: 1G; FIBER: 0G; PROTEIN: 0G; SUGAR: 0G; SWEETENER CARBS: 4G

# HOT TODDY

The hot toddy is a warm, soothing beverage, often touted as a cold remedy for stuffy heads and sore throats. It's light, pleasant, and restorative, much like a relaxing cup of tea. Honey is used in more traditional hot toddies, but sugar-free honey-flavored extracts and low-carb simple syrup work to lower the carb content. Enjoy when you're feeling under the weather, when the temperature drops outside, or to treat your friends during the holiday season.

¾ cup water

1½ ounces whiskey

½ ounce Low-Carb Simple Syrup (page 116)

2 teaspoons freshly squeezed lemon juice

⅛ teaspoon sugar-free honey flavor extract (see Prep Tip, page 51)

1 cinnamon stick, for garnish (optional)

TOOLS: small saucepan or tea kettle, Irish coffee mug or heat-resistant glassware, jigger, citrus squeezer, bar spoon

Bring the water to a simmer in a small saucepan over medium-high heat. Once simmering, carefully pour the hot water into a mug. Add the whiskey, simple syrup, lemon juice, and honey extract. Stir gently and serve garnished with a stick of cinnamon (if using).

VARIATION: Maple syrup is often used as a replacement for honey in this cocktail. Though traditional maple syrup is not suitable for keto, there are loads of sugar-free maple-flavored syrups available to choose from. Mix in 2 to 3 teaspoons of maple flavoring instead of the honey flavoring and low-carb simple syrup.

PER SERVING: CALORIES: 99; TOTAL FAT: 0G; TOTAL CARBOHYDRATES: 1G; FIBER: 0G; PROTEIN: 0G; SUGAR: 0G; SWEETENER CARBS: 8G

# CASANOVA

This cocktail has multiple variations; some are brandy-based whereas others are built with whiskey, and they couldn't be any more different! The brandy cocktail calls for orange juice, bitters, ginger, and cayenne pepper, whereas the bourbon drink is rich with cream, Kahlúa, and sweet Marsala, a fortified wine. To make the whiskey version low in carbs, use homemade low-carb coffee liqueur in lieu of Kahlúa and replace the sweet Marsala with dry red wine.

1½ ounces bourbon

1 ounce heavy cream

¾ ounce dry red wine

¾ ounce Low-Carb Coffee
   Liqueur (page 118)

---

TOOLS: shaker, jigger, strainer, cocktail glass (chilled)

Fill a shaker with ice and add the bourbon, cream, wine, and coffee liqueur. Shake well and strain into a cocktail glass.

> VARIATION: Unsweetened coconut cream or a dairy-free milk can be used in place of the heavy cream if needed. Consider unflavored almond, coconut, and hemp seed milk as alternatives.

PER SERVING: CALORIES: 237; TOTAL FAT: 11G; TOTAL CARBOHYDRATES: 2G; FIBER: 0G; PROTEIN: 1G; SUGAR: 1G; SWEETENER CARBS: 6G

# IRISH COFFEE

This cocktail is frequently confused with coffee mixed with Baileys Irish Cream liqueur. Sure, that concoction is a delicious after-dinner drink, but it's not Irish Coffee. To make a true Irish Coffee, you spike the brewed coffee with Irish whiskey, then mix in brown sugar or maple syrup, and top with whipped cream. It's the whiskey that adds "Irish" to the cocktail's name, not the Irish cream liqueur. To reduce carbs, here we use maple extract and low-carb simple syrup to replace the usual sweeteners.

2 ounces heavy whipping cream

4 ounces freshly brewed hot coffee

1½ ounces Irish whiskey

½ ounce Low-Carb Simple Syrup (page 116)

2 or 3 drops maple extract (optional)

TOOLS: medium bowl, electric mixer or whisk, Irish coffee mug, jigger, bar spoon

Pour the cream into a medium bowl and, using an electric mixer, whisk on medium for 3 to 4 minutes, until soft peaks form. Fill a mug with the hot coffee. Add the whiskey, simple syrup, and maple extract (if using) and stir well. Carefully float the whipped cream on top. Serve immediately.

VARIATION: To make an iced Irish coffee, use cold brew instead. Fill a glass with ice, cold brew coffee, whiskey, simple syrup, and maple extract. Top with the whipped cream, then stir the ingredients together with a bar spoon.

PER SERVING: CALORIES: 293; TOTAL FAT: 21G; TOTAL CARBOHYDRATES: 2G; FIBER: 0G; PROTEIN: 1G; SUGAR: 2G; SWEETENER CARBS: 8G

# DRY ROB ROY

This a variation of the Manhattan (page 103), made with Scotch instead of rye whiskey. To keep carbs down, use dry vermouth or dry white wine and skip the maraschino cherries. Simple alterations like these can build new low-carb drinks. For example, adding low-carb simple syrup makes it similar to a Flying Scotsman. And replacing the Angostura with orange bitters is comparable to a Highland Fling. Using a dry red wine in place of vermouth is like an Affinity.

2½ ounces Scotch

½ ounce dry vermouth or dry white wine

1 dash Angostura bitters

Lemon twist, for garnish

TOOLS: old-fashioned glass, mixing glass, jigger, strainer, bar spoon, paring knife

Fill a glass with ice. Fill a mixing glass with ice and add the Scotch, vermouth, and bitters. Stir well and strain into the glass. Finish with a lemon twist to garnish.

> PREP TIP: You can also serve this drink "up" instead, straining it into a chilled cocktail glass without ice.

PER SERVING: CALORIES: 183; TOTAL FAT: 0G; TOTAL CARBOHYDRATES: 2G; FIBER: 0G; PROTEIN: 0G; SUGAR: 0G; SWEETENER CARBS: 0G

# WHISKEY SOUR

Another old-school classic, this is an impressive little drink for how simple it is. The citrusy tang of the freshly squeezed lemon juice plays off the low-key sweetness perfectly, yin to the yang. The cleverly balanced flavor offers an ideal opportunity to dress up a budget whiskey, but higher-quality spirits won't go to waste. Many prefer the cocktail with bourbon, but don't let that stop you from mixing in your whiskey of choice. Serve the drink "up" or on the rocks.

2½ ounces bourbon

1 ounce freshly squeezed lemon juice

½ ounce Low-Carb Simple Syrup (page 116)

Lemon slice, for garnish

TOOLS: shaker, jigger, citrus squeezer, strainer, sour glass or cocktail glass (chilled), paring knife

Fill a shaker with ice and add the bourbon, lemon juice, and simple syrup. Shake well and strain into a glass. Garnish with a lemon slice.

VARIATION: Though the whiskey sour is excellent as is, the cocktail has inspired numerous variations building on the classic base. If you add dry red wine, that's a New York Sour. Shake it with an egg white, and you'll get a Boston Sour. Mix in some peppermint flavoring for a Stinger Sour. Or sneak in a bit of gin for a Park Lane.

PER SERVING: CALORIES: 161; TOTAL FAT: 0G; TOTAL CARBOHYDRATES: 2G; FIBER: 0G; PROTEIN: 0G; SUGAR: 1G; SWEETENER CARBS: 8G

# MANHATTAN

Though the Prohibition-era classic is rich with sugar from sweet vermouth and a maraschino cherry, this dry version is perfectly suitable for keto. Dry vermouth replaces the sweet variety, naturally reducing carbs. If you'd prefer to reduce carbs further, opting for a dry white wine in place of the vermouth will do the job.

2 ounces rye whiskey

¾ ounce dry vermouth or dry white wine

3 dashes Angostura bitters

Lemon twist, for garnish

TOOLS: mixing glass, jigger, strainer, bar spoon, cocktail glass (chilled), paring knife

Fill a mixing glass with ice and add the whiskey, vermouth, and bitters and stir well. Strain into a glass and twist the lemon over the drink, wipe the rim with the lemon, and drop it into the glass.

PREP TIP: The whiskey used to make a Manhattan significantly influences the flavor of the drink, so feel free to use whatever type you prefer. Rye, bourbon, and blended Canadian whiskey are most commonly used. However, Scotch and Irish whiskey are also popular.

PER SERVING: CALORIES: 163; TOTAL FAT: 0G; TOTAL CARBOHYDRATES: 3G; FIBER: 0G; PROTEIN: 0G; SUGAR: 0G; SWEETENER CARBS: 0G

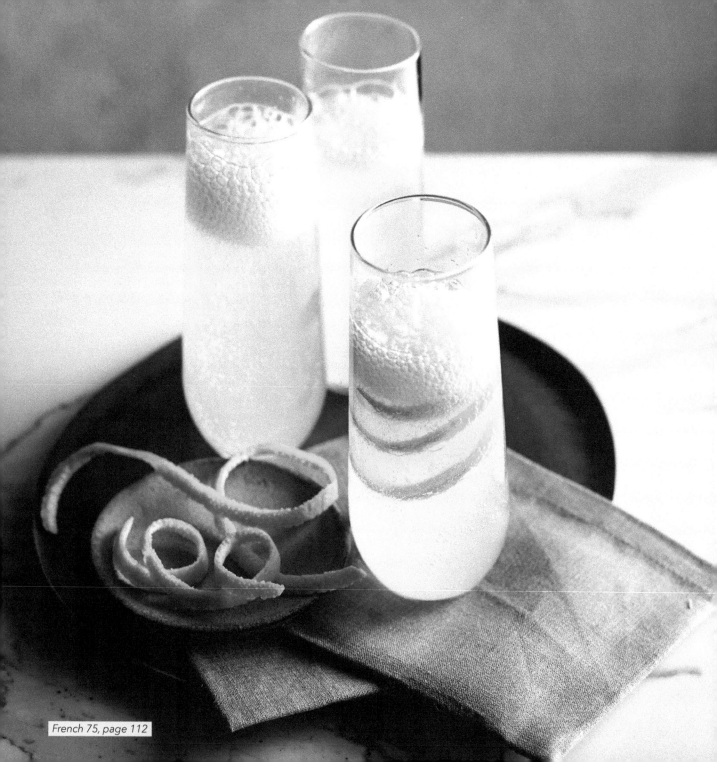

French 75, page 112

# = **10** =
## PUNCHES, SHOOTERS, LIQUEURS, AND MIXED SPIRITS

# BRASS MONKEY

This legendary cocktail was made famous by the Beastie Boys' song of the same name. If you've ever wondered what the song was about, they're simply handing out lessons on how to serve this drink (and the subsequent aftermath). According to the lyrics, you can drink it anytime or anyplace (or pour it on your face). Orange juice is traditional, but orange-flavored sparkling water provides a lower-carb mixer.

1 ounce vodka

¾ ounce light rum

½ ounce Low-Carb Simple Syrup (page 116)

⅛ teaspoon anise extract or licorice extract/flavoring (optional)

4 ounces orange-flavored sparkling water

TOOLS: highball glass, jigger, bar spoon

Fill a glass with ice. Add the vodka, rum, simple syrup, and anise extract (if using) and stir well. Top with orange-flavored sparkling water and unleash your inner Beastie Boy.

VARIATION: Though orange-flavored sparkling water is similar in many ways to orange juice, it's not quite the same as freshly squeezed OJ. Adding an ounce of fresh orange juice can kick up the flavor, though it will spike the carbs a bit (3.2g per ounce). A lower-carb alternative for the bright citrus acidity is an ounce of freshly squeezed lemon juice (2.1g per ounce).

PER SERVING: CALORIES: 113; TOTAL FAT: 0G; TOTAL CARBOHYDRATES: 0G; FIBER: 0G; PROTEIN: 0G; SUGAR: 0G; SWEETENER CARBS: 8G

# GELATIN SHOOTERS

**MAKES 20 SHOOTERS**

The key to making gelatin shooters hold up well is a proper ratio of liquid to gelatin. For every 0.3 ounce of gelatin mix, you will need 1 cup of boiling water and 1 cup of chilled liquid. The chilled liquid could be vodka, champagne, your favorite spiked seltzer, a low-carb liqueur, or whatever your heart desires.

2 cups water

2 mint sprigs (optional)

1 (0.3-ounce) package sugar-free strawberry gelatin mix (or flavor of choice)

½ cup water or hard seltzer, chilled

½ cup vodka or booze of choice, chilled

**TOOLS:** small saucepan or tea kettle, heatproof bowl, whisk, 2-ounce party cups, rimmed baking sheet

Heat the water and mint (if using) in a small saucepan or kettle until boiling. Remove the mint sprigs and measure 1 cup of the water. Whisk with the gelatin mix in a heatproof bowl for 2 minutes. (Discard the remaining hot water.) Allow the gelatin mixture to cool for about 5 minutes. Whisk in the chilled water, then the chilled vodka. Place 20 (2-ounce) disposable party cups on a rimmed baking sheet, then fill each with the gelatin mixture. Refrigerate for a minimum of 4 hours to set, and store refrigerated until ready to serve, or up to 1 week tightly covered.

> **PREP TIP:** Unflavored gelatin and sweetener can be used if you prefer making your flavors with different ingredients, such as muddled berries, citrus, extracts, or water flavorings. Replace each 0.3-ounce packet of gelatin mix with 2 teaspoons of unflavored gelatin.

**PER SERVING (1 SHOOTER):** CALORIES: 13; TOTAL FAT: 0G; TOTAL CARBOHYDRATES: 0G; FIBER: 0G; PROTEIN: 0G; SUGAR: 0G; SWEETENER CARBS: 0G

# ALABAMA SLAMMER

This cocktail traditionally uses sugary, high-carb liqueurs, including Southern Comfort, amaretto, and sloe gin. Here, whiskey replaces the Southern Comfort, while juniper berry flavor extract and gin replace the sloe gin to achieve a similar flavor profile with reduced carbs. Also known as a Southern Slammer, it's often served as a shooter-style drink, but it's certainly tasty enough to be a sipping cocktail. Serve on the rocks or "up," but don't feel obligated to slam it because of the name.

1 ounce whiskey

1 ounce Homemade Amaretto (page 119)

½ ounce Low-Carb Simple Syrup (page 116)

¼ ounce gin

⅛ teaspoon juniper berry flavor extract

1 dash freshly squeezed lemon juice

**TOOLS:** highball glass, shaker, jigger, citrus squeezer, strainer

Fill a glass with ice. Fill a shaker with ice and add the whiskey, amaretto, simple syrup, gin, juniper extract, and lemon juice. Shake well and strain into the glass.

**VARIATION:** The juniper berry flavor extract replicates the flavors found in sloe gin liqueur, but other berry extracts and water flavorings can make tasty alternatives.

**PER SERVING:** CALORIES: 112; TOTAL FAT: 0G; TOTAL CARBOHYDRATES: 0G; FIBER: 0G; PROTEIN: 0G; SUGAR: 0G; SWEETENER CARBS: 13G

# TIGER'S MILK

Although it may sound exotic, and despite its relative obscurity, this is a top-notch cocktail. If you enjoy a drink in the style of a White Russian (page 82), you will absolutely love this recipe. Traditionally, the drink calls for half-and-half and simple syrup, but low-carb simple syrup and diluted heavy cream slash a significant number of carbs from the recipe.

3 ounces water

1 ounce brandy

1 ounce rum

1 ounce heavy cream

½ ounce Low-Carb Simple Syrup (page 116)

Nutmeg, ground or grated, for garnish

TOOLS: shaker, jigger, strainer, wine glass or highball glass (chilled)

Fill a shaker with ice and add the water, brandy, rum, cream, and simple syrup. Shake vigorously and strain into a glass. Sprinkle the nutmeg on top to garnish.

PREP TIP: Serve the drink on the rocks if preferred: Just strain the liquid into a glass filled with ice.

PER SERVING: CALORIES: 227; TOTAL FAT: 11G; TOTAL CARBOHYDRATES: 1G; FIBER: 0G; PROTEIN: 1G; SUGAR: 1G; SWEETENER CARBS: 8G

# MULLED CIDER

**MAKES 10 DRINKS**

Although the apple cider traditionally used here is high in carbohydrates, sugar-free spiced apple drink mixes or herbal tea can replicate the flavors of this cold-weather classic. Whole cloves and cinnamon sticks infuse the cocktail with the quintessential warm spices that make this drink perfect for chilly winter days. Whether it's spiked or booze-free, mulled cider is a favorite at holiday gatherings.

10 cups water

5 (4-gram) pouches sugar-free spiced apple cider mix or apple spice herbal tea bags

½ cup crystallized allulose or sweetener of choice

2 lemon slices

10 whole cloves

2 cinnamon sticks

2 cups brandy

**TOOLS:** large pot, mixing spoon, large heatproof bowl, ladle, heatproof glasses or mugs

Combine the water, apple cider mix, allulose, lemon slices, cloves, and cinnamon sticks in a large pot and bring to a simmer over medium heat. Reduce the heat to low and simmer for about 10 minutes, stirring periodically. Pour in the brandy and stir briefly. Remove from the heat and carefully transfer the mixture to a heatproof serving bowl (discard the tea bags if herbal tea was used). Ladle the liquid into heatproof glassware to serve.

> **VARIATION:** If cider isn't to your liking, you can opt for mulled wine instead by trading the water and spiced apple ingredients for two bottles of dry red wine. You can keep the brandy or leave it out.

**PER SERVING:** CALORIES: 103; TOTAL FAT: 0G; TOTAL CARBOHYDRATES: 0G; FIBER: 0G; PROTEIN: 0G; SUGAR: 0G; SWEETENER CARBS: 6G

# AMARETTO SOUR

Amaretto sours are often made by mixing a sweet almond-flavored liqueur with a premade sweet and sour mix. The resulting drink is sugary and high in carbs. This rendition employs a homemade amaretto and freshly squeezed lemon juice. The traditional maraschino cherry garnish is also swapped out for a lower-carb alternative: blueberry and lemon.

2 ounces Homemade Amaretto (page 119)

1 ounce freshly squeezed lemon juice

1 blueberry, for garnish

Lemon slice, thinly cut, for garnish

---

TOOLS: shaker, jigger, citrus squeezer, strainer, sour glass or cocktail glass (chilled), paring knife, cocktail skewer

Fill a shaker with ice and add the amaretto and lemon juice. Shake vigorously and strain into a glass. Thread the blueberry and lemon slice onto a cocktail skewer and balance it across the glass's lip for garnish.

VARIATION: If you prefer a frothy Amaretto Sour, dry shake (without ice) the liquid ingredients with an egg white. Add ice and give the drink an additional shake before straining into a glass. This step will leave a thick, foamy layer on top of the beverage.

PER SERVING: CALORIES: 72; TOTAL FAT: 0G; TOTAL CARBOHYDRATES: 2G; FIBER: 0G; PROTEIN: 0G; SUGAR: 0G; SWEETENER CARBS: 10G

# FRENCH 75

Aptly named after a war weapon, this is not your typical champagne brunch fare. You can't tell by looking at it, but this sparkling glass of bubbly is remarkably potent and can be a bit dangerous. The gin provides an unexpected punch that will knock you flat if you aren't careful. Serve when you want to turn brunch into a full-on rager or to kickstart Sunday Funday.

1 ounce gin

½ ounce freshly squeezed lemon juice

½ ounce Low-Carb Simple Syrup (page 116)

4 ounces brut or extra-brut champagne, chilled

Orange peel spiral, (see page 23) for garnish

**TOOLS:** shaker, jigger, citrus squeezer, strainer, champagne flute (chilled) or Collins glass, paring knife

Fill a shaker with ice and add the gin, lemon juice, and simple syrup. Shake well and strain into a chilled champagne flute or ice-filled glass. Top with the champagne and garnish with an orange peel spiral.

> **PREP TIP:** Choose your glassware based on whether you are serving the drink "up" or on the rocks. If you are serving without ice, go for a chilled champagne glass. If you prefer it with ice, a tall Collins glass works better.

**PER SERVING:** CALORIES: 146; TOTAL FAT: 0G; TOTAL CARBOHYDRATES: 4G; FIBER: 0G; PROTEIN: 0G; SUGAR: 1G; SWEETENER CARBS: 8G

# JUNIPER ROYALE

This cocktail is made keto-friendly by exchanging regular cranberry juice for diet, swapping grenadine for pomegranate water flavoring, and choosing the driest champagne. An opportunity to trim carbs even further lies in the orange juice: You can either use less of it or trade it out for orange-flavored sparkling water. Thanks to the fizzy champagne, this cocktail is perfect for celebrations, but it's also a great low-carb replacement for the brunch-time mimosa.

1 ounce gin

1 ounce diet
cranberry juice

½ ounce fresh
orange juice

1 teaspoon pomegranate
water flavoring or
⅛ teaspoon juniper
berry flavor extract

3 ounces brut or extra-brut
champagne, chilled

**TOOLS:** shaker, jigger,
citrus squeezer, strainer,
champagne flute (chilled),
bar spoon

Fill a shaker with ice and add the gin, cranberry juice, orange juice, and pomegranate flavoring. Shake well and strain into a glass. Top with the champagne and slowly stir.

**PREP TIP:** Be careful not to add the champagne to the shaker when preparing the drink. Shaking champagne is like shaking up a soda; it will lose all effervescence and fall flat. Keep your bubbly full of bubbles and reserve the champagne for a top-off directly into the glass.

**PER SERVING:** CALORIES: 149; TOTAL FAT: 0G; TOTAL CARBOHYDRATES: 4G; FIBER: 0G; PROTEIN: 0G; SUGAR: 1G; SWEETENER CARBS: 6G

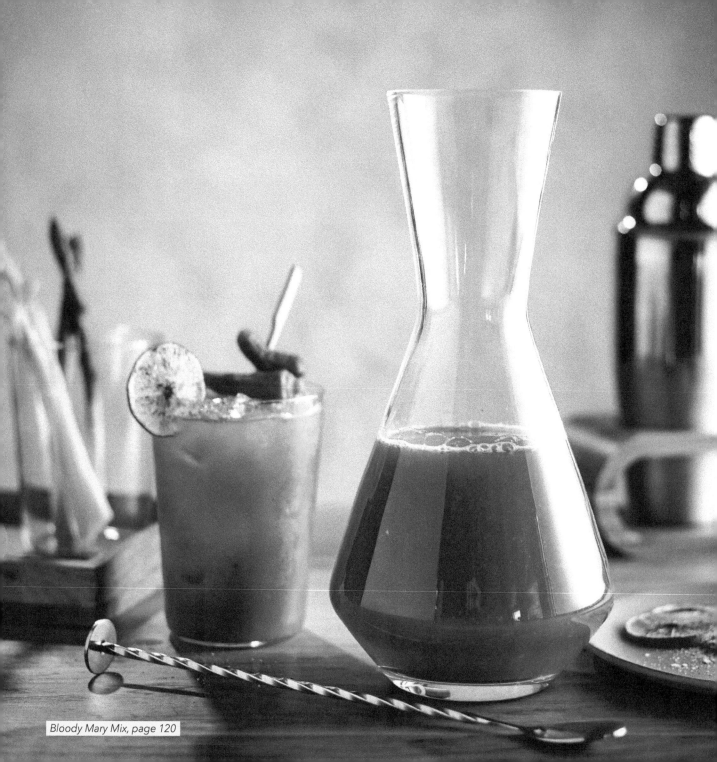

*Bloody Mary Mix, page 120*

# = 11 =
# SYRUPS, MIXERS, AND FLAVORINGS

# LOW-CARB SIMPLE SYRUP (WITH VARIATIONS)

**MAKES ¾ CUP**

This keto-friendly simple syrup is a staple component in over one-quarter of the cocktail recipes in this book. I prefer using crystallized allulose, which rivals the consistency of traditional simple syrup, but you can use whichever sweetener you prefer, using the conversion ratios on page 169.

½ cup water

½ cup crystallized allulose or sweetener of choice

TOOLS: small saucepan, whisk, sealable 8-ounce glass bottle or jar, funnel (optional)

Combine the water and allulose in a small saucepan and whisk over medium heat until the sweetener dissolves, about 1 minute. Remove from the heat and cool to room temperature. Carefully transfer the mixture to a glass storage bottle or jar. Seal the container and store in the refrigerator for up to 2 months. Reseal tightly after each use.

> **VARIATIONS**
>
> ORANGE-FLAVORED SYRUP (TRIPLE SEC SUBSTITUTE): Add 1 tablespoon of orange extract.
>
> MINT SYRUP: Add 1 tablespoon of mint extract or steep fresh mint leaves in the syrup.
>
> HERB OR SPICE SYRUP: Steep fresh or dried herb leaves, seeds, or whole spices directly in the mixture. Try rosemary, thyme, basil, fennel, cardamom, ginger, cinnamon, chamomile tea, lemongrass, lavender, pepper, anise, chile, and so on.

**PER SERVING (1 OUNCE):** CALORIES: 0; TOTAL FAT: 0G; TOTAL CARBOHYDRATES: 0G; FIBER: 0G; PROTEIN: 0G; SUGAR: 0G; SWEETENER CARBS: 5G

# LOW-CARB ORANGE LIQUEUR

**MAKES 2¾ CUPS**

This recipe is the keto-friendly answer to Cointreau, Grand Marnier, Curaçao, and any other orange liqueur you may encounter in traditional cocktails. The classic liqueurs differ based on where and how the oranges are sourced, aged, and processed, but as a time- and carb-saver, I often skip the oranges and use flavor extract instead. If you'd prefer to stick with fresh citrus, see the Variation that follows.

2 cups vodka

1 tablespoon orange flavor extract

½ cup crystallized allulose or sweetener of choice

½ cup water

**TOOLS:** sealable 24-ounce glass bottle or jar, funnel (optional), small saucepan, whisk

Combine the vodka and orange extract in a glass bottle or jar. Combine the allulose and water in a small saucepan and whisk over medium heat until the sweetener dissolves, about 1 minute. Remove from the heat and cool to room temperature. Carefully transfer the syrup to the glass container. Seal the container and store refrigerated for up to 2 months. Tightly reseal after each use.

**VARIATION:** Orange liqueur starts with a spirit infused with orange peels (the sugar comes later). So if you want to skip the orange extract in a cocktail, you can make your own orange-flavored vodka. Steep orange peels directly in vodka for 2 weeks, then strain the vodka through cheesecloth or a fine-mesh sieve. It's a bit more time-consuming, but the flavors are worth the wait!

**PER SERVING (1 OUNCE):** CALORIES: 47; TOTAL FAT: 0G; TOTAL CARBO-HYDRATES: 0G; FIBER: 0G; PROTEIN: 0G; SUGAR: 0G; SWEETENER CARBS: 5G

# LOW-CARB COFFEE LIQUEUR

**MAKES 5¼ CUPS**

This coffee liqueur is a keto-friendly Kahlúa copycat. The flavor is indistinguishable from the classic, but unlike the traditional liqueur, there is hardly any sugar to speak of. The vanilla bean will need to steep for several days, so be sure to account for this step in your prep time, or try the shortcut in the tip!

2 cups unsweetened cold brew coffee, or hot-brewed coffee cooled to room temperature

1½ cups rum or vodka

1 vanilla bean, halved lengthwise

1 cup water

1½ cups crystallized allulose or sweetener of choice

**TOOLS:** sealable 48-ounce glass bottle or jar, funnel (optional), small saucepan, whisk

Place the coffee, rum, and vanilla bean in a glass bottle or jar. Combine the water and allulose in a small saucepan and whisk over medium heat until the sweetener dissolves, about 1 minute. Remove from the heat and cool to room temperature. Carefully transfer the syrup to the glass container. Seal the container and store in the refrigerator for 3 to 4 days, then remove the vanilla bean. Reseal the container and store in the refrigerator for up to 2 months.

> **PREP TIP:** If you prefer a more instant version of the recipe, skip steeping the vanilla bean and opt for 1 tablespoon of vanilla extract instead.

**PER SERVING (1 OUNCE):** CALORIES: 24; TOTAL FAT: 0G; TOTAL CARBOHYDRATES: 0G; FIBER: 0G; PROTEIN: 0G; SUGAR: 0G; SWEETENER CARBS: 9G

# HOMEMADE AMARETTO

**MAKES 3½ CUPS**

Amaretto is a famous Italian liqueur with a distinct almond flavor. It's a foundational component in many drinks, including the Amaretto Sour (page 111) and Alabama Slammer (page 108), but it's very high in carbs. Luckily, you can make your own and achieve matching flavors with simple, convenient ingredients—things you likely have in your cabinets already. If you don't have almond extract, you can swap it for an additional 2 tablespoons of vanilla extract.

1 cup water

1 cup crystallized allulose or sweetener of choice

2 cups vodka

2 tablespoons almond extract

1 tablespoon maple extract

2 teaspoons vanilla extract

**TOOLS:** small saucepan, whisk, sealable 32-ounce glass bottle or jar, funnel (optional)

Combine the water and allulose in a small saucepan over medium heat and whisk until the sweetener dissolves, about 1 minute. Remove from the heat and cool to room temperature. When the syrup is cool to the touch, stir in the vodka and almond, maple, and vanilla extracts. Carefully transfer the mixture to a glass storage container. Seal tightly and store refrigerated for up to 2 months.

**VARIATION:** Many homemade amaretto recipes call for both white and brown sugar. If you choose to use a low-carb brown sugar substitute, use ½ cup of brown sugar substitute with ½ cup of crystallized allulose to sweeten the recipe, and omit the maple extract.

**PER SERVING (1 OUNCE):** CALORIES: 32; TOTAL FAT: 0G; TOTAL CARBOHYDRATES: 0G; FIBER: 0G; PROTEIN: 0G; SUGAR: 0G; SWEETENER CARBS: 5G

# BLOODY MARY MIX

**MAKES 6½ CUPS**

It's certainly possible to build individual Bloody Marys from scratch, but if you're serving up a crowd, it's more practical to have a big batch of mix ready to go. Tomato juice is often used as the mixer base, but here, diluted tomato paste flavors the drink and reduces the carbs. You can add or change ingredients to make unique blends. Soy sauce, mustard, vinegar, pickle or olive brine, ginger, and wasabi are all popular ingredient choices that work well. For the way I serve a Bloody Mary, see page 90.

6 cups water

1 (6-ounce) can tomato paste

2 tablespoons Worcestershire sauce

1 tablespoon onion powder

2 garlic cloves, peeled

1 teaspoon celery salt

TOOLS: blender, large pitcher

Add the water, tomato paste, Worcestershire sauce, onion powder, garlic, and celery salt to a blender and puree until smooth. Place the blender pitcher in the refrigerator until ready to serve, or transfer the mixture to a large serving pitcher.

PREP TIP: Because of the large volume of water used in this recipe, you will need a blender that can accommodate at least 48 fluid ounces. If you don't have a large enough blender available, you can halve the recipe for smaller batches or use a handheld immersion blender in a large pot to mix the full quantity.

PER SERVING (½ CUP): CALORIES: 15; TOTAL FAT: 0G; TOTAL CARBOHYDRATES: 3G; FIBER: 1G; PROTEIN: 1G; SUGAR: 2G; SWEETENER CARBS: 0G

# MARGARITA MIX

MAKES 3½ CUPS

Although it may be tempting to grab a premade margarita mixer out of convenience, you wouldn't be doing yourself any favors. The processed mixers have loads of sugar, and they don't taste that great. Crafting your own mixers will always yield better results—carbs or not. This batch recipe has an uncomplicated preparation that can be easily scaled up or down to the desired number of servings.

1 cup freshly squeezed lemon juice

½ cup freshly squeezed lime juice

1½ cups water

1 cup crystallized allulose or sweetener of choice

TOOLS: citrus squeezer, sealable 32-ounce glass bottle or jar, small saucepan, whisk, funnel (optional)

Combine the lemon and lime juices in a glass bottle or jar. Combine the water and allulose in a small saucepan over medium heat and whisk until the sweetener dissolves, about 1 minute. Remove from the heat and cool to room temperature. Carefully transfer the syrup to the bottle. Seal the container and shake well to mix. Store refrigerated for up to 2 months and tightly reseal after each use.

PREP TIP: To prepare a keto-friendly margarita, shake 3 ounces of the margarita mix with 2 ounces of tequila in an ice-filled shaker. Or blend the drink with ½ cup of ice. Serve in a glass rimmed with lime juice and salt.

PER SERVING (3 OUNCES): CALORIES: 10; TOTAL FAT: 0G; TOTAL CARBO-HYDRATES: 3G; FIBER: 0G; PROTEIN: 0G; SUGAR: 1G; SWEETENER CARBS: 24G

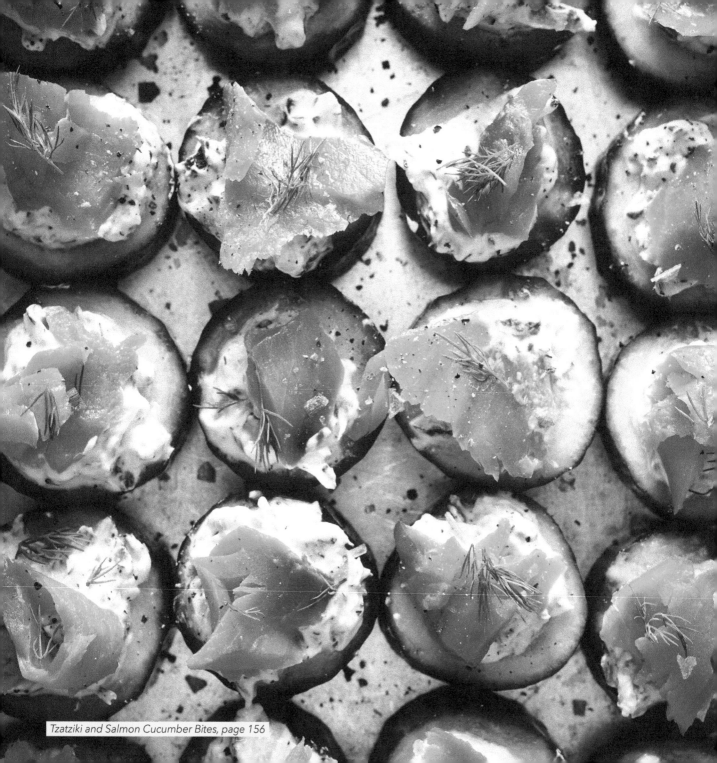

Tzatziki and Salmon Cucumber Bites, page 156

# = 12 =
# HAPPY HOUR MUNCHIES

# RED HOT CHILI-GARLIC WINGS

**SERVES 4 | PREP TIME: 15 MINUTES / COOK TIME: 1 HOUR**

**DAIRY-FREE, GLUTEN-FREE, NUT-FREE**

No happy hour is complete without hot wings. These baked chicken wings deliver a potent blend of chili and garlic without overwhelming your taste buds with spiciness. If you prefer more of a kick, serve the chicken with extra chili-garlic sauce or sambal paste for dipping.

3 tablespoons Thai chili-garlic sauce or sambal oelek chili paste

2 tablespoons avocado oil or extra-virgin olive oil

2 teaspoons onion powder

1 garlic clove, minced

12 chicken wings, separated at the joint

½ teaspoon salt

½ teaspoon freshly ground black pepper

2 scallions, both green and white parts, sliced, for garnish

1. Preheat the oven to 375°F. Line a rimmed baking sheet with parchment paper or aluminum foil and set aside.

2. In a resealable bag, combine the chili-garlic sauce, oil, onion powder, and garlic. Add the wings to the bag, seal, and shake until well coated.

3. Arrange the wings on the baking sheet in a single layer and sprinkle with the salt and pepper.

4. Bake for 1 hour, or until crispy and fully cooked, turning once halfway through. Remove from the oven and serve garnished with the sliced scallions.

> **STORAGE TIP:** Store the wings in an airtight container in the refrigerator for up to 4 days.

**PER SERVING (3 WINGS):** CALORIES: 685; TOTAL FAT: 49G; TOTAL CARBO-HYDRATES: 2G; FIBER: 1G; PROTEIN: 56G; SUGAR: 0G; SWEETENER CARBS: 0G

**MACROS:** FAT: 64%; PROTEIN: 35%; CARBS: 1%

# STEAK BITES WITH ROASTED RED PEPPER SAUCE

**SERVES 4 | PREP TIME: 15 MINUTES / COOK TIME: 5 MINUTES**

**GLUTEN-FREE, NUT-FREE** ——————————————————

Are you searching for a sure-fire way to impress guests without spending excess time in the kitchen? Look no further. This recipe is done in a matter of minutes and elevates a boring budget steak to rave-worthy status. To save on prep time, look for precut "beef tips" at your local grocery store or butcher counter.

### FOR THE STEAK

1 pound sirloin steak, trimmed of fat and gristle, cut into 1-inch cubes

¼ teaspoon salt

¼ teaspoon freshly ground black pepper

2 tablespoons unsalted butter, divided

### TO MAKE THE STEAK

1. Season the steak cubes with the salt and pepper.

2. In a large skillet, melt 1 tablespoon of butter over medium-high heat. Once the butter begins to brown, working in batches, add the steak to the skillet in a single layer. Cook without stirring or flipping for 30 to 45 seconds, then flip the pieces over with a spatula and cook for an additional 30 to 45 seconds. This will sear the outside but keep the inside medium-rare.

3. Transfer to a clean plate and repeat the process with the remaining butter and steak cubes.

CONTINUED >>

**FOR THE SAUCE**

1 (12-ounce) jar roasted red bell peppers, drained

½ cup extra-virgin olive oil

2 tablespoons freshly squeezed lemon juice

1 garlic clove, peeled

½ teaspoon dried basil

¼ teaspoon salt

¼ teaspoon freshly ground black pepper

**TO MAKE THE SAUCE**

4. In a food processor, combine the roasted red peppers, oil, lemon juice, garlic, basil, salt, and pepper and process until smooth. Transfer the sauce to four small bowls for dipping. Serve immediately with the steak bites.

> **STORAGE TIP:** Store leftovers in an airtight container in the refrigerator for up to 4 days.

**PER SERVING:** CALORIES: 528; TOTAL FAT: 46G; TOTAL CARBOHYDRATES: 5G; FIBER: 1G; PROTEIN: 23G; SUGAR: 3G; SWEETENER CARBS: 0G

**MACROS:** FAT: 78%; PROTEIN: 19%; CARBS: 3%

# HANGOVER HOMIES

**SERVES 2 | PREP TIME: 10 MINUTES / COOK TIME: 15 MINUTES**

**GLUTEN-FREE, NUT-FREE, VEGETARIAN**

A popular brunch menu item with the same name from a local cafe bar inspired this recipe, which is a powerhouse breakfast packed with nourishing ingredients to help you battle the worst of it. Eggs, avocado, and scallions sit atop a mountain of keto home fries to banish headaches and settle your stomach after a night of overindulgence. Of course, you can enjoy this meal any time— it's delicious even when you feel like a million bucks.

1 tablespoon avocado oil

1 large turnip, peeled (if desired) and diced

1 tablespoon minced onion

4 large eggs, lightly beaten

¼ cup sour cream

¼ cup shredded cheddar cheese

½ avocado, peeled, pitted, and sliced

Pinch salt

Pinch freshly ground black pepper

1 scallion, both green and white parts, chopped

1. In a large skillet, heat the oil over medium-high heat. Add the turnip and onion and cook, stirring frequently, until tender, 12 to 15 minutes.

2. Meanwhile, warm a nonstick skillet over medium heat. Pour in the eggs and pull them from side to side with a spatula as they cook to form soft curds. Remove from the heat when the egg is no longer visibly runny. Evenly divide the cooked eggs between two plates.

3. When the turnip mixture is done, add it to the eggs, dividing evenly.

4. In a small bowl, mix the sour cream and cheddar, then add to the eggs and turnips.

CONTINUED >>

5. Divide the avocado between the plates and season with salt and pepper. Garnish with the scallion. Serve immediately.

> **PREP TIP:** If you prefer fried eggs, crack them directly into the hot pan and cook, covered, until the whites set. Remove from the heat for sunny-side up, or flip and cook for an additional 1 to 5 minutes for over-easy to over-hard.

**PER SERVING:** CALORIES: 439; TOTAL FAT: 34G; TOTAL CARBOHYDRATES: 15G; FIBER: 6G; PROTEIN: 19G; SUGAR: 7G; SWEETENER CARBS: 0G

**MACROS:** FAT: 70%; PROTEIN: 18%; CARBS: 12%

# BACON AND BLUE CHEESE STUFFED JALAPEÑOS

**MAKES 24 JALAPEÑOS | PREP TIME: 15 MINUTES / COOK TIME: 15 MINUTES**

**GLUTEN-FREE, NUT-FREE**

Is it even a party without a platter of jalapeños loaded with ooey-gooey cheese? These are a terrific appetizer for a crowd. Serve them up for game day, a barbecue, a potluck, or just a back porch happy hour. Any excuse to make these is a good one!

6 bacon slices

8 ounces cream cheese, at room temperature

½ cup crumbled blue cheese

1 teaspoon onion powder

1 teaspoon garlic powder

Pinch salt

Pinch freshly ground black pepper

12 jalapeño peppers, halved lengthwise and seeded

1. Preheat the oven to 400°F. Line a rimmed baking sheet with parchment paper or aluminum foil and set aside.

2. In a large skillet, cook the bacon over medium-high heat until the fat renders, about 10 minutes. Transfer to a plate lined with paper towels to cool, then crumble.

3. In a medium bowl, mix the bacon, cream cheese, blue cheese, onion powder, garlic powder, salt, and pepper.

4. Fill the hollow of each jalapeño half with the bacon and cheese mixture and arrange cut-side up on the baking sheet. Bake for 15 minutes, rotating the sheet halfway through. Remove from the oven and transfer to a serving platter.

**STORAGE TIP:**
Store leftovers in an airtight container in the refrigerator for up to 4 days.

**PER SERVING (2 JALAPEÑO HALVES):** CALORIES: 75; TOTAL FAT: 7G; TOTAL CARBOHYDRATES: 1G; FIBER: 0G; PROTEIN: 3G; SUGAR: 1G; SWEETENER CARBS: 0G

**MACROS:** FAT: 78%; PROTEIN: 15%; CARBS: 7%

# COCONUT SHRIMP DIPPERS

**SERVES 6 | PREP TIME: 15 MINUTES / COOK TIME: 15 MINUTES**

**DAIRY-FREE, GLUTEN-FREE**

Skip the played-out shrimp cocktail and whip up some of these dippers for your next get-together instead. The peanut dipping sauce and coconut flavors are a match made in heaven, but if peanut or nut allergens are a concern, consider an alternative dip, such as a citrus-infused mayo with fresh lemon or lime juice.

## FOR THE SHRIMP

Coconut oil cooking spray

½ cup coconut flour

1 teaspoon freshly ground black pepper

2 large eggs

½ cup unsweetened coconut flakes

⅓ cup crushed pork rinds

30 large shrimp, peeled and deveined, tails left on

## TO MAKE THE SHRIMP

1. Preheat the oven to 425°F. Mist a rimmed baking sheet with coconut oil and set aside.

2. Prepare three shallow bowls for dredging: In the first bowl, combine the coconut flour and pepper. In the second bowl, beat the eggs. In the third bowl, mix the coconut flakes and crushed pork rinds. Line the bowls up in the same order, with the prepped baking sheet at the end. Dip each shrimp into the flour mixture, then into the egg, then into the coconut flake mixture. Place the coated shrimp on the baking sheet. Continue until all the shrimp are dredged, then mist the tops of the shrimp with coconut oil.

3. Bake the shrimp for 10 minutes, then flip and continue baking for an additional 5 to 6 minutes, until the shrimp are fully cooked.

½ cup unsweetened peanut butter or almond butter

½ cup tamari or coconut aminos

¼ cup water

1 tablespoon red curry paste

1 teaspoon Thai chili-garlic sauce (optional)

## TO MAKE THE SAUCE

4. In a bowl, stir together the peanut butter, tamari, water, curry paste, and chili-garlic sauce (if using) until smooth. Transfer to a group serving bowl or individually portioned dishes.

5. Serve the shrimp with the sauce for dipping.

> **STORAGE TIP:** Leftovers can be stored in an airtight container in the refrigerator for up to 3 days.

**PER SERVING:** CALORIES: 317; TOTAL FAT: 17G; TOTAL CARBOHYDRATES: 13G; FIBER: 7G; PROTEIN: 28G; SUGAR: 4G; SWEETENER CARBS: 0G

**MACROS:** FAT: 48%; PROTEIN: 35%; CARBS: 17%

# LOADED CHAYOTE CURLY FRIES

**SERVES 4 | PREP TIME: 10 MINUTES / COOK TIME: 30 MINUTES**

**GLUTEN-FREE, NUT-FREE**

I'm crazy about chayote squash and firmly believe it to be the unsung hero of low-carb vegetables. Chayote is a pale-green, pear-shaped veggie common in Latin American cuisine, and offers so much versatility on its own or as a dietary swap, including as a potato substitute. If you can't find chayote squash, you can also make these fries with turnips, though the flavor will be slightly earthy.

4 bacon slices

4 chayote squash

1 tablespoon extra-virgin olive oil or avocado oil

½ teaspoon salt

⅛ teaspoon freshly ground black pepper

½ cup shredded cheddar cheese

4 scallions, both green and white parts, sliced

1. Preheat the oven to 425°F. Line a rimmed baking sheet with parchment paper or aluminum foil and set aside.

2. In a medium skillet, cook the bacon over medium-high heat until the fat renders, about 10 minutes. Transfer to a plate lined with paper towels to cool, then crumble.

3. Use a vegetable peeler to strip the skin from the chayote squash. Rinse the sticky coating from the peeled squash. Spiralize the chayote into curly shapes. Or, if you don't have a spiralizer, cut the squash into ¼-inch-thick fry-style wedges. Discard any remnants of the center seeds. Toss the chayote with the oil, salt, and pepper, then spread on the baking sheet in a single layer.

4. Roast for 15 minutes for curly fries or 20 minutes for wedges, or until tender and browned.

5. Remove the fries from the oven and adjust the temperature setting to broil. Sprinkle the cheddar evenly over the top and return to the oven. Broil for 1 to 2 minutes, until the cheese has melted.

6. Sprinkle the bacon and scallions over the top. Serve immediately.

**PER SERVING:** CALORIES: 175; TOTAL FAT: 12G; TOTAL CARBOHYDRATES: 11G; FIBER: 4G; PROTEIN: 8G; SUGAR: 4G; SWEETENER CARBS: 0G

**MACROS:** FAT: 61%; PROTEIN: 17%; CARBS: 22%

> STORAGE TIP:
> Store leftovers in an airtight container in the refrigerator for up to 3 days.

# SEA SALT AND VINEGAR ZUCCHINI CHIPS

**SERVES 4 | PREP TIME: 20 MINUTES, PLUS 2 HOURS TO MARINATE / COOK TIME: 2 HOURS**

**DAIRY-FREE, GLUTEN-FREE, NUT-FREE, VEGAN**

The key to making zucchini chips is a low temperature and slow cooking time. In this recipe, the oven ensures crispy vegetables, but a dehydrator will also do the job. To save time, consider using a premixed salt and vinegar seasoning instead of soaking the zucchini in vinegar.

2 large zucchini, thinly sliced crosswise (see Prep Tip)

½ cup apple cider vinegar

1 tablespoon extra-virgin olive oil

1 teaspoon sea salt

1. Place the sliced zucchini in a shallow glass dish and cover with the vinegar. Let it marinate in the refrigerator for a minimum of 2 hours or overnight.

2. Once marinated, lay out sheets of paper towel and place the drained zucchini on them in a single layer. Cover with additional paper towels and set a weighted baking sheet on top to remove excess moisture.

3. Preheat the oven to 235°F. Line two rimmed baking sheets with parchment paper and lightly brush each with some of the oil.

4. Arrange the zucchini slices closely together on the baking sheets but in a single layer. Brush them with the rest of the oil and sprinkle with the salt.

5. Bake for 2 hours, without flipping, until crisp and golden. If some zucchini slices cook faster than others, remove the crisp slices and allow the damp ones to bake longer. Transfer the finished zucchini from the pans to fresh, dry paper towels to cool. Serve.

> **PREP TIP:** To ensure the zucchini chips cook evenly, use a sharp knife or (ideally) a mandoline to cut the discs to uniform thickness.

**PER SERVING:** CALORIES: 64; TOTAL FAT: 4G; TOTAL CARBOHYDRATES: 5G; FIBER: 2G; PROTEIN: 2G; SUGAR: 3G; SWEETENER CARBS: 0G

**MACROS:** FAT: 60%; PROTEIN: 8%; CARBS: 32%

# BUFFALO CHICKEN QUESADILLAS

**SERVES 4 | PREP TIME: 15 MINUTES / COOK TIME: 35 MINUTES**

**GLUTEN-FREE, NUT-FREE**

The tortillas for these quesadillas are made with coconut flour, which is highly absorbent, so be sure to check the consistency of the batter before pouring it into the skillet. If it's too thick, the mixture will be difficult to work with. Consider using store-bought low-carb tortillas as a time-saver.

## FOR THE TORTILLAS

2 large eggs

10½ tablespoons unsweetened coconut milk beverage or unsweetened almond milk, divided

8 teaspoons coconut flour

1 teaspoon unflavored gelatin powder or psyllium husk powder

Extra-virgin olive oil, for greasing the pan

## TO MAKE THE TORTILLAS

1. In a large bowl, whisk together the eggs, 6½ tablespoons of coconut milk, and the coconut flour until the batter is smooth.

2. In a small bowl, combine the remaining 4 tablespoons of coconut milk and gelatin powder and let sit for 5 minutes. Whisk the gelatin mixture until smooth, without clumps, then pour into the coconut flour batter and whisk to combine. The batter should be a liquid, pourable consistency. If it's too thick, add additional coconut milk, 1 tablespoon at a time, until the batter is thin enough to pour and easily spread over the pan.

3. Lightly coat a medium nonstick skillet with oil and warm over medium heat. Pour one-quarter of the batter (about ¼ cup) into the hot skillet and swirl to distribute the mixture and coat the bottom of the pan as you would when making omelets or crepes. Cover with a lid and cook

### FOR THE FILLING

2 tablespoons extra-virgin olive oil

1 large boneless, skinless chicken breast

1 cup shredded cheddar cheese

¼ cup Buffalo hot sauce

> **STORAGE TIP:** Store leftover quesadillas in an airtight container in the refrigerator for up to 1 day. Tortillas can be stored in an airtight container in the refrigerator for up to 2 weeks.

for 2 minutes. Flip the tortilla, cover, and cook for an additional 2 minutes. Transfer to a clean plate. Repeat to make a total of 4 tortillas.

### TO MAKE THE FILLING

4. In a large skillet, heat the oil over medium-high heat. Add the chicken breast and cook for 4 to 5 minutes per side, turning once, until no longer pink. Remove from the heat. When cool enough to handle, shred or dice.

5. In a large bowl, combine the cooked chicken, cheddar, and Buffalo hot sauce.

6. Set the nonstick skillet over medium-low heat. Lay one of the tortillas in the skillet. Spread one-quarter of the chicken mixture (about ½ cup) on half of the tortilla, then fold the other side over the top. Cover with a lid and cook for 1 minute, then flip, cover, and cook for another minute, or until the cheese has melted. Remove from the heat. Repeat to make a total of four quesadillas. Cut into triangle wedges and serve immediately.

**PER SERVING:** CALORIES: 267; TOTAL FAT: 17G; TOTAL CARBOHYDRATES: 9G; FIBER: 2G; PROTEIN: 20G; SUGAR: 2G; SWEETENER CARBS: 0G

**MACROS:** FAT: 57%; PROTEIN: 30%; CARBS: 13%

# PRETZEL BITES WITH MUSTARD CHEESE SAUCE

**SERVES 6 | PREP TIME: 25 MINUTES / COOK TIME: 10 MINUTES**

**GLUTEN-FREE, VEGETARIAN**

These pretzel bites are made using a variation of the infamous "Fat Head pizza" base, a surprisingly versatile low-carb dough recipe made primarily from melted cheese. Naturally, there is an ungodly amount of dairy here—if you don't play well with lactose or other milk components, it's best to steer clear. The dough is forgiving and can be easily mixed and kneaded by hand, but feel free to use a stand mixer with a dough hook attachment if you prefer.

**FOR THE PRETZELS**

1 tablespoon warm water

1 teaspoon active
  dry yeast

½ cup almond flour

1 large egg

1 cup shredded
  low-moisture
  mozzarella cheese

2 tablespoons
  cream cheese

1 tablespoon unsalted
  butter, melted

¼ teaspoon coarse salt

**TO MAKE THE PRETZELS**

1. Preheat the oven to 400°F. Line a rimmed baking sheet with parchment paper or a silicone baking mat and set aside.

2. In a large bowl, mix the water with the yeast and let rest for 5 to 10 minutes, until the yeast rehydrates. Add the almond flour and egg and whisk to combine.

3. In a microwave-safe bowl, microwave the mozzarella and cream cheese in 30-second intervals, stirring with a fork, until the cheese is soft, pliable, and fully melted together. Transfer the melted cheese to the bowl with the yeast mixture and use a fork to mix until thoroughly combined.

1 tablespoon
  unsalted butter

¼ cup heavy cream

¼ cup shredded
  cheddar cheese

½ teaspoon
  mustard powder

¼ teaspoon freshly ground
  black pepper

⅛ teaspoon fine salt

4. Divide the dough into four equal portions. Lay a sheet of parchment paper on the work surface. Wet your hands with warm water and roll one dough portion into a long rope about 1 inch in diameter. Cut the dough into 1-inch lengths and place them on the baking sheet. Repeat with the remaining dough.

5. Brush the tops of the dough pieces with the melted butter and sprinkle with the salt. Bake for 10 to 12 minutes, until golden brown.

## TO MAKE THE CHEESE SAUCE

6. Meanwhile, in a small saucepan, melt the butter over medium heat. Whisk in the cream and bring to a boil, then remove from the heat. Stir in the cheddar, mustard powder, pepper, and salt until smooth and thoroughly combined. Transfer to a serving dish.

7. Serve the pretzel bites with the cheese sauce for dipping.

> PREP TIP: Work quickly with the dough mixture, as it will be sticky and begin to harden if left at room temperature for long. If the dough does begin to solidify, briefly reheat it in the microwave for several seconds. Periodically wet your hands with warm water to prevent the dough from sticking.

PER SERVING: CALORIES: 221; TOTAL FAT: 19G; TOTAL CARBOHYDRATES: 4G; FIBER: 1G; PROTEIN: 9G; SUGAR: 1G; SWEETENER CARBS: 0G

MACROS: FAT: 77%; PROTEIN: 17%; CARBS: 7%

# ALMOST-ZERO CARB CHEESEBURGERS

**SERVES 4 | PREP TIME: 15 MINUTES / COOK TIME: 20 MINUTES**

**GLUTEN-FREE, NUT-FREE**

Bunless burgers are all the rage on keto. But I, much like Sir Mix-a-Lot, like big buns and I cannot lie. So this recipe has instructions for making stupid-simple hamburger buns along with fresh, juicy burger patties. You can dress them up however you like, though the condiments suggested here will keep the carbs for an entire cheeseburger just a hair above zero.

**FOR THE BUNS**

¾ cup egg whites (from about 6 large eggs)

½ teaspoon baking powder

½ teaspoon xanthan gum

1 (30-gram) scoop unsweetened unflavored whey protein powder

1 teaspoon ground flaxseed

¼ teaspoon sesame seeds

**TO MAKE THE BUNS**

1. Preheat the oven to 350°F. Line a rimmed baking sheet with parchment paper or a silicone baking mat and set aside.

2. In a large bowl, with an electric mixer, beat the egg whites, baking powder, and xanthan gum on medium for 7 to 8 minutes, until stiff peaks form.

3. In a small bowl, mix the protein powder and ground flaxseed together, then gently fold into the egg white mixture. Scoop four separate mounds of the mixture onto the baking sheet. Sprinkle the sesame seeds over the top.

4. Bake for 15 to 20 minutes, until golden brown. Remove from the oven to cool, then slice the rolls in half horizontally.

1 pound ground beef

¼ teaspoon salt

¼ teaspoon freshly ground
black pepper

1 tablespoon
unsalted butter

4 cheddar cheese slices

FOR ASSEMBLY

1 tablespoon mayonnaise

1 tablespoon
yellow mustard

1 dill pickle, sliced

## TO MAKE THE BURGERS

5. Meanwhile, in a large bowl, combine the ground beef, salt, and pepper. Divide the meat into four portions and form into 1-inch-thick patties with the palms of your hand or a burger press. Use your fingers to press a shallow dimple in the center of each patty.

6. In a large skillet, melt the butter over medium heat, then increase the heat to medium-high. Place the patties in the hot pan without crowding them. Cook for 3 to 4 minutes, then flip and top with the cheddar slices. Cook for another 3 to 4 minutes, until the burgers reach your preferred doneness.

## TO ASSEMBLE

7. Dress the buns with a thin layer of mayonnaise and mustard. Place the patties on the bottom half of the buns and top with pickle slices. Top with the buns and serve immediately.

PER SERVING: CALORIES: 508; TOTAL FAT: 38G; TOTAL CARBOHYDRATES: 3G; FIBER: 0G; PROTEIN: 36G; SUGAR: 1G; SWEETENER CARBS: 0G

MACROS: FAT: 68%; PROTEIN: 29%; CARBS: 3%

# CAPRESE SKEWERS

**MAKES 12 SKEWERS | PREP TIME: 15 MINUTES**

**GLUTEN-FREE, NUT-FREE, VEGETARIAN** —————————————————

Everyone loves a caprese salad, but serving it on a skewer makes it much easier to nibble while mingling. The ingredient ratios are adapted to be lower in carbs while still maintaining the quintessential flavor profile. Note that tomatoes don't last as long once they have been cut. Be conservative with how many skewers you prepare; leftovers do not store well.

48 fresh basil leaves

18 cherry
  tomatoes, halved

24 small fresh
  mozzarella balls

1 tablespoon
  balsamic vinegar

⅛ teaspoon salt

1. Onto each of 12 wooden skewers, thread 4 basil leaves, 3 cherry tomato halves, and 2 mozzarella balls, alternating as you go.

2. Lay the skewers flat on a serving tray and drizzle the balsamic vinegar in a zigzag pattern over the top. Season with the salt and serve immediately or store refrigerated in an airtight container for up to 1 day.

**PER SERVING (2 SKEWERS):** CALORIES: 41; TOTAL FAT: 2G; TOTAL CARBO-HYDRATES: 3G; FIBER: 1G; PROTEIN: 3G; SUGAR: 2G; SWEETENER CARBS: 0G

**MACROS:** FAT: 50%; PROTEIN: 25%; CARBS: 25%

# BURRATA-STUFFED MUSHROOMS

**MAKES 20 MUSHROOMS | PREP TIME: 15 MINUTES / COOK TIME: 15 MINUTES**

**GLUTEN-FREE, NUT-FREE, VEGETARIAN**

Stuffed mushrooms are a cocktail party staple and an undisputed crowd-pleaser. If your usual mushroom fillings start to feel a bit humdrum and unimaginative, switch it up with burrata. Burrata has a firm mozzarella shell with a cream and soft-curd filling. It's wonderful baked, but if you prefer the cheese fresh, try baking the mushroom caps alone and adding the stuffing afterward.

20 cremini mushroom caps, cleaned

1 tablespoon extra-virgin olive oil

¼ cup chopped arugula, divided

6 ounces fresh burrata cheese or fresh mozzarella, at room temperature, cut or torn into 20 even-size chunks

5 cherry tomatoes, quartered

¼ teaspoon flaky sea salt

¼ teaspoon freshly ground black pepper

1. Preheat the oven to 425°F. Line a rimmed baking sheet with parchment paper or aluminum foil.

2. On the prepared baking sheet, toss the mushroom caps in the oil and place them gill-side up. Distribute half of the arugula evenly among the mushrooms. Place a burrata chunk in each cap, followed by a cherry tomato quarter. Sprinkle the salt, pepper, and remaining arugula over the tops of the stuffed mushrooms.

3. Bake for 15 to 20 minutes, until the mushrooms are tender. Transfer to a platter and serve immediately.

**PER SERVING (2 MUSHROOMS):** CALORIES: 73; TOTAL FAT: 5G; TOTAL CARBOHYDRATES: 2G; FIBER: 1G; PROTEIN: 5G; SUGAR: 1G; SWEETENER CARBS: 0G

**MACROS:** FAT: 64%; PROTEIN: 27%; CARBS: 9%

# KETO-FRIENDLY CHARCUTERIE BOARD

**SERVES 10 | PREP TIME: 15 MINUTES**

**GLUTEN-FREE**

Charcuterie boards, or antipasto platters, are a popular option for keto entertaining. This recipe only scratches the surface for potential ingredient combinations, as there are so many possibilities! Consider adding pickled vegetables, changing up the nuts and cheese, or choosing other low-sugar fruits. You can also fill the board with homemade appetizers, like the Salami and Cream Cheese Pinwheels (page 154), Olive Tapenade "Crostini" (page 152), or the Spinach-Artichoke Dip (page 157).

½ cup small fresh mozzarella balls

½ cup halved strawberries

½ cup raspberries

½ cup green olives or olives of choice, pitted

¼ cup whole almonds

1. Choose a large flat serving platter that can comfortably hold all the ingredients in your desired arrangement. Place the mozzarella, strawberries, raspberries, olives, and almonds in small separate bowls. Set the containers on the platter spaced apart.

- ½ cup cheddar cheese cubes
- 4 ounces pepper Jack cheese, thinly sliced
- 4 ounces Swiss cheese, thinly sliced
- 4 ounces prosciutto, thinly sliced
- 4 ounces hard salami, thinly sliced
- 6 bacon slices, cooked and halved
- 4 ounces turkey, thinly sliced

2. Begin arranging the remaining meats and cheeses around the bowls, adjusting aesthetics as you fill the space. Start near the dishes, working out and away from the bowl to tightly fill the empty space on the platter in a single layer. If necessary, stack the ingredients upward. Tuck ingredients in empty spaces, fan-out, roll, and fold items if necessary. Serve immediately or cover and store in the refrigerator until ready to serve.

STORAGE TIP: Store leftovers in an airtight container in the refrigerator for up to 1 week.

PER SERVING: CALORIES: 263; TOTAL FAT: 19G; TOTAL CARBOHYDRATES: 4G; FIBER: 1G; PROTEIN: 18G; SUGAR: 1G; SWEETENER CARBS: 0G

MACROS: FAT: 64%; PROTEIN: 30%; CARBS: 6%

# VEGGIE LOVER CRUDITÉS PLATTER

**SERVES 10 | PREP TIME: 30 MINUTES**

**GLUTEN-FREE, NUT-FREE, VEGETARIAN**

Prepackaged crudités make for a convenient, no-effort keto party platter. The downside? They can be a little boring, especially compared to some high-carb treats competing for attention at most get-togethers. Do all your vegetable-loving friends a favor and whip up a veggie platter that will blow all the other snacks out of the water.

1 cup mayonnaise

1 cup sour cream or plain Greek yogurt

1 teaspoon onion powder

Generous pinch salt

Generous pinch freshly ground black pepper

½ cup cucumber slices, cut at an angle

½ cup celery sticks (4 inches long)

½ cup quartered radishes

½ cup cherry tomatoes

½ cup broccoli florets

½ cup cauliflower florets

½ cup snap peas

½ cup orange bell pepper strips

1. Choose one or two large flat serving platters that can comfortably hold several cups of cut vegetables and dips in your desired arrangement.

2. In a small bowl, combine the mayonnaise, sour cream, onion powder, salt, and pepper. Transfer the dip to one or two clean serving bowls (depending on the number of platters) and swirl the top. Place a bowl near the center of each serving platter.

½ cup whole pickled banana peppers

2 Belgian endives, leaves separated

1 cup Kalamata olives or mixed olive varieties, pitted

3. Begin arranging the vegetables, adjusting for aesthetics as you fill the space. Start near the dip(s), working out and away from the bowl to tightly fill the empty space on the platter with the vegetables. Tuck ingredients into empty spaces and fan out items as necessary. Serve immediately.

> PREP TIP: Cut up your veggies no more than 2 hours before guests arrive so they will be nice and crisp.

PER SERVING: CALORIES: 227; TOTAL FAT: 23G; TOTAL CARBOHYDRATES: 5G; FIBER: 2G; PROTEIN: 2G; SUGAR: 2G; SWEETENER CARBS: 0G

MACROS: FAT: 89%; PROTEIN: 3%; CARBS: 8%

# GLAZED COCKTAIL MEATBALLS

**SERVES 6 | PREP TIME: 10 MINUTES / COOK TIME: 35 MINUTES**

**DAIRY-FREE, GLUTEN-FREE, NUT-FREE** ─────────────────

Most cocktail meatball recipes call for a grape jelly coating and use processed frozen meatballs packed with fillers and extra carbs. Using fresh ingredients and ditching the jelly dramatically reduces the carbs while boosting the flavor. These meatballs can be enjoyed on their own or used for a unique component on a Keto-Friendly Charcuterie Board (page 144).

8 ounces ground pork

8 ounces ground beef

½ cup shredded zucchini, drained

1 large egg

1 garlic clove, minced

1¼ teaspoons salt, divided

¼ teaspoon freshly ground black pepper, divided

1 (6-ounce) can tomato paste

¼ cup crystallized allulose or sweetener of choice

2 tablespoons apple cider vinegar

1. Preheat the oven to 325°F. Line a rimmed baking sheet with aluminum foil and place a wire rack on top.

2. In a large bowl, combine the pork, beef, zucchini, egg, garlic, ¾ teaspoon of salt, and ⅛ teaspoon of pepper using your hands. Pull off tablespoon-size portions and roll into balls. Set on the rack.

3. Bake for 20 minutes. (The meatballs will not be fully cooked through yet.)

4. In a large saucepan, combine the tomato paste, allulose, vinegar, remaining ½ teaspoon of salt, and remaining ⅛ teaspoon of pepper. Bring to a simmer over medium heat and simmer for 5 minutes. Reduce the heat to low.

5. Add the parbaked meatballs to the pan and cook for an additional 10 minutes, gently stirring to coat the meatballs thoroughly.

6. Transfer the meatballs to a serving platter and serve with toothpicks. Or, place in a slow cooker on a low setting to keep the meatballs warm until serving.

> **STORAGE TIP:** Store leftovers in an airtight container in the refrigerator for up to 1 week.

**PER SERVING:** CALORIES: 234; TOTAL FAT: 16G; TOTAL CARBOHYDRATES: 6G; FIBER: 1G; PROTEIN: 15G; SUGAR: 4G; SWEETENER CARBS: 8G

**MACROS:** FAT: 64%; PROTEIN: 27%; CARBS: 9%

# FRIED MAC 'N' CHEESE BALLS

**MAKES 12 BALLS | PREP TIME: 30 MINUTES, PLUS 3 HOURS TO CHILL /
COOK TIME: 20 MINUTES**

GLUTEN-FREE

This dish is inspired by one my partner and I ate at a dive bar in an old bowling alley. We'd been eyeing the daily special when our waitress appeared. We asked if it was any good. She nodded and said, "I know a guy," before disappearing into the back. She returned with drinks and a sizzling basket of deep-fried macaroni and cheese. Best. Bar food. Ever. To lower the carbs, cauliflower is used in place of macaroni noodles, and the breading consists of pork rinds and almond meal.

1 tablespoon extra-virgin olive oil

1 head cauliflower, cut into ½-inch pieces

2 tablespoons cubed cream cheese

½ cup heavy cream

¼ teaspoon xanthan gum

1 cup shredded cheddar cheese

½ teaspoon salt

¼ teaspoon smoked paprika

1 cup avocado oil

½ cup finely crushed pork rinds

½ cup almond flour

1 large egg

1. In a large skillet, heat the olive oil over medium heat. Add the cauliflower and sauté for 10 minutes, or until tender.

2. In a medium saucepan, melt the cream cheese over medium-low heat. Increase the heat to medium, whisk in the heavy cream and xanthan gum, and bring to a boil. Remove from the heat and whisk in the cheddar until smooth. Stir in the salt and smoked paprika.

3. Pour the cheese mixture over the cauliflower and stir well. Allow to cool, then chill in the refrigerator for 3 hours, or until firm.

4. In a large cast-iron skillet or small Dutch oven, heat the avocado oil over medium-high heat until hot enough to sizzle a crumb of bread dropped in it.

5. Set up a dredging station: Combine the pork rinds and almond flour in one bowl. Beat the egg in a second bowl. Scoop the cheesy cauliflower mixture into 1-inch balls. Dip the balls into the egg, then dredge in the pork-rind mixture until fully coated.

6. Working in batches, place the balls in the hot oil and cook for 2 to 3 minutes, until crispy. Transfer to paper towels to drain and cool slightly. Serve immediately.

**PER SERVING (1 BALL):** CALORIES: 156; TOTAL FAT: 15G; TOTAL CARBOHYDRATES: 3G; FIBER: 1G; PROTEIN: 5G; SUGAR: 1G; SWEETENER CARBS: 0G

**MACROS:** FAT: 80%; PROTEIN: 14%; CARBS: 6%

# OLIVE TAPENADE "CROSTINI"

**SERVES 6 | PREP TIME: 15 MINUTES / COOK TIME: 35 MINUTES**

**GLUTEN-FREE, NUT-FREE, VEGETARIAN** ⸻

Think you need to be a skilled baker to whip up a homemade baguette and crostini? Think again. If you can beat egg whites with an electric mixer, you can tackle this crostini recipe with ease. The olive tapenade is even simpler, requiring only a few quick pulses in a food processor. Make the bread and tapenade to serve together, or enjoy either separately.

### FOR THE CROSTINI

- ¾ cup egg whites (from about 6 large eggs)
- ½ teaspoon baking powder
- ½ teaspoon xanthan gum
- 1 (30-gram) scoop unsweetened, unflavored whey protein powder
- 2 tablespoons extra-virgin olive oil
- ⅛ teaspoon salt

### TO MAKE THE CROSTINI

1. Preheat the oven to 350°F. Line a rimmed baking sheet with parchment paper or a silicone baking mat and set aside.

2. In a large bowl, with an electric mixer, combine the egg whites, baking powder, and xanthan gum and beat on medium for 7 to 8 minutes, until stiff peaks form. Gently fold the protein powder into the egg white mixture. Scoop the mixture onto the baking sheet into 2 long, thin log-shaped mounds (like baguettes).

3. Bake for 20 to 25 minutes, until crisp and golden brown. Remove from the oven. Leave the oven on and increase the temperature to 375°F.

4. When the baguettes are cool, use a serrated knife to cut each loaf crosswise into ¼-inch-thick slices.

## FOR THE TAPENADE

1 cup Kalamata olives or mixed olive varieties, pitted

¼ cup fresh basil leaves

2 tablespoons extra-virgin olive oil

2 tablespoons capers

1 tablespoon freshly squeezed lemon juice

1 garlic clove, peeled

Pinch salt

Pinch freshly ground black pepper

5. Lightly brush both sides of each piece with the oil and lay the slices flat on the baking sheet. Sprinkle the tops with the salt. Bake for 5 minutes, then flip the crostini and bake for an additional 5 minutes. Remove from the oven and transfer to a rack to cool.

### TO MAKE THE TAPENADE

6. In a food processor, combine the olives, basil leaves, oil, capers, lemon juice, garlic, salt, and pepper and pulse until the desired consistency is reached. Scrape down the sides between pulses. Several pulses yield a relish-like texture, while more pulsing creates a spreadable sauce.

7. Spoon the tapenade onto the prepared crostini and serve immediately.

**PER SERVING:** CALORIES: 141; TOTAL FAT: 11G; TOTAL CARBOHYDRATES: 4G; FIBER: 1G; PROTEIN: 7G; SUGAR: 0G; SWEETENER CARBS: 0G

**MACROS:** FAT: 71%; PROTEIN: 19%; CARBS: 10%

# SALAMI AND CREAM CHEESE PINWHEELS

**SERVES 8 | PREP TIME: 15 MINUTES**

**GLUTEN-FREE, NUT-FREE**

These pinwheels are superb on their own, but make an impressive addition to a Keto-Friendly Charcuterie Board (page 144). Plastic wrap is essential for making this dish from start to finish, so be sure you have plenty to spare before getting started.

1 (8-ounce) block cream cheese

8 ounces deli-style hard salami, thinly sliced

1 tablespoon chopped arugula

2 scallions, both green and white parts, chopped

1. Lay a large piece of plastic wrap on a work surface and smooth out any wrinkles. Place the block of cream cheese in the center. Cover with a second sheet of plastic wrap and, using a rolling pin, roll it into a thin (about ¼ inch thick) rectangle.

2. Remove the top piece of plastic wrap and cover the cheese with a layer of overlapping salami slices, in a fashion similar to roof tiling. When the cream cheese is fully covered and no longer visible, place a fresh layer of plastic wrap over the top. Flip the wrapped salami and cheese so that the cream cheese side is facing up. Remove the top piece of plastic wrap and sprinkle the arugula and scallions evenly over the cream cheese.

3. Starting from a long side, tightly roll the salami up and over the cream cheese (as you would a jelly roll) until you meet the other long side to form a log with the salami surface on the outside. Wrap the log tightly with plastic wrap, securing each end by twisting the wrap. Roll the wrapped log over the work surface to smooth out any trapped pockets of air within the log. Chill in the refrigerator until ready to serve.

4. To serve, remove the plastic wrap and use a very sharp knife to cut crosswise into ¼-inch-thick slices. Place on a platter and serve.

**PER SERVING:** CALORIES: 205; TOTAL FAT: 19G; TOTAL CARBOHYDRATES: 2G; FIBER: 0G; PROTEIN: 7G; SUGAR: 1G; SWEETENER CARBS: 0G

**MACROS:** FAT: 81%; PROTEIN: 16%; CARBS: 3%

STORAGE TIP: Store any leftovers in an airtight container in the refrigerator for up to 4 days.

# TZATZIKI AND SALMON CUCUMBER BITES

**SERVES 6 | PREP TIME: 30 MINUTES**

**GLUTEN-FREE, NUT-FREE**

These cucumber bites are light and refreshing, the perfect combo for cocktail party finger food. Cucumber retains a lot of water, so don't skip the draining process described below to prevent fluid from pooling in the cut area.

2½ large cucumbers, divided

½ cup plain Greek yogurt

1½ tablespoons chopped fresh dill, divided

1½ teaspoons freshly squeezed lemon juice

1 garlic clove, minced

Pinch salt

Pinch freshly ground black pepper

4 ounces smoked salmon, cut into thin strips

1. Trim the ends from the 2 whole cucumbers and cut into about 24 (¾-inch-thick) discs. Use a melon baller or spoon to scoop out a ½-inch-deep well in the center of each disc. Place the cucumbers on paper towels to drain excess moisture.

2. Finely grate the half cucumber onto a paper towel. Wrap the cucumber in the towel and squeeze out excess moisture. Place the grated cucumber in a large bowl. Add the yogurt, 1 tablespoon of dill, lemon juice, garlic, salt, and pepper and mix to combine.

3. Fill each cucumber cup with the tzatziki sauce. Top each cucumber with a strip of smoked salmon and garnish all the cups with the remaining ½ tablespoon of dill. Place on a serving dish and serve immediately.

**PER SERVING:** CALORIES: 54; TOTAL FAT: 2G; TOTAL CARBOHYDRATES: 6G; FIBER: 1G; PROTEIN: 5G; SUGAR: 3G; SWEETENER CARBS: 0G

**MACROS:** FAT: 26%; PROTEIN: 36%; CARBS: 38%

# SPINACH-ARTICHOKE DIP

**SERVES 6 | PREP TIME: 10 MINUTES / COOK TIME: 15 MINUTES**

GLUTEN-FREE, NUT-FREE, VEGETARIAN ————

So often, premixed seasoning packets and ready-made dressings are packed with sugar, despite their savory flavors. Making your own batches of dips, sauces, and condiments from scratch puts you in charge of the carb count. It's easy enough and tastes a whole lot better, too. Enjoy this dip with fresh veggies or on "Crostini" (page 152).

1 tablespoon extra-virgin olive oil

¼ medium onion, diced

1 (10-ounce) package frozen chopped spinach, thawed and drained

1 (14-ounce) can artichoke hearts, drained and chopped

1 garlic clove, minced

8 ounces cream cheese, at room temperature

¼ cup grated Parmesan cheese

1 cup plain Greek yogurt or sour cream

¼ cup mayonnaise

Pinch salt

Pinch freshly ground black pepper

1. In a large saucepan, heat the oil over medium-high heat. Add the onion and cook until translucent, about 10 minutes. Add the spinach, artichokes, and garlic and sauté for 3 to 5 minutes, until the spinach and artichokes are tender.

2. Reduce the heat to medium-low and stir in the cream cheese and Parmesan until melted. Remove from the heat and stir in the yogurt and mayonnaise until thoroughly combined. Season with salt and pepper.

3. Serve as a dip or a spread.

> STORAGE TIP: Store in an airtight container in the refrigerator for up to 2 weeks.

PER SERVING: CALORIES: 341; TOTAL FAT: 31G; TOTAL CARBOHYDRATES: 10G; FIBER: 4G; PROTEIN: 8G; SUGAR: 3G; SWEETENER CARBS: 0G

MACROS: FAT: 81%; PROTEIN: 8%; CARBS: 11%

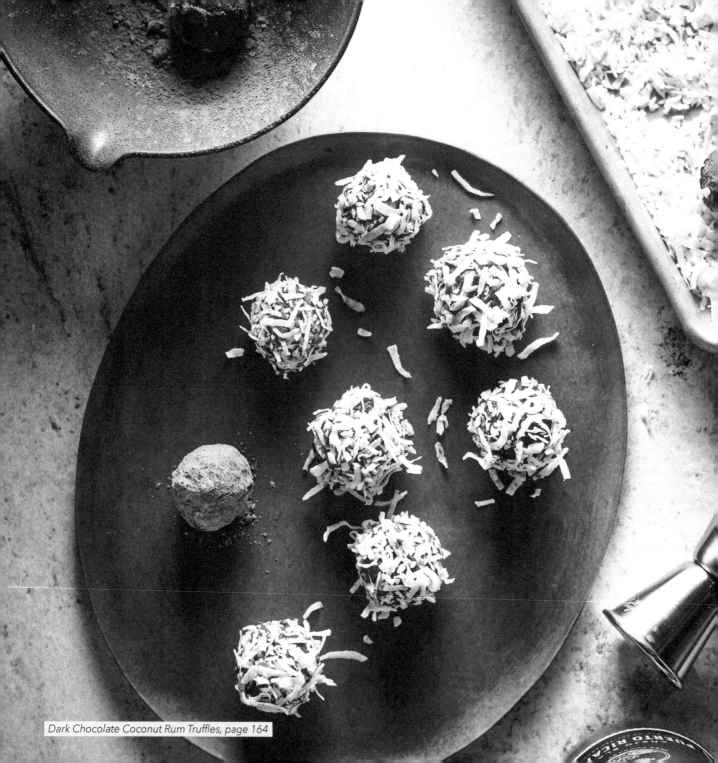

*Dark Chocolate Coconut Rum Truffles, page 164*

# = 13 =
# DESSERTS AND SWEET TREATS

# DRUNKEN GUMMY BEARS

**MAKES ABOUT 150 GUMMIES | PREP TIME: 15 MINUTES, PLUS 2 HOURS TO SET /
COOK TIME: 10 MINUTES**

**DAIRY-FREE, GLUTEN-FREE, NUT-FREE**

Scrap the traditional vodka-soaked candy and infuse homemade gummies with wine instead. The beauty of making your own candy is that you can go from sugar-filled to sugar-free with a few minor tweaks. Consider experimenting with champagne, hard spirits, and flavor extracts to suit your preferences.

2 cups dry red, white, or rosé wine, at room temperature, divided

¼ cup unflavored gelatin powder

¾ cup crystallized allulose or sweetener of choice

1 drop food coloring (optional)

1. Place silicone gummy bear molds on a baking sheet. In a small bowl, combine 1 cup of wine and the gelatin, stir well, and allow to sit undisturbed for several minutes.

2. In a medium saucepan, simmer the remaining 1 cup of wine over medium heat until the volume is reduced by half, about 10 minutes. Remove from the heat. Whisk the allulose and gelatin mixture into the hot wine until completely dissolved. Add the food coloring (if using).

3. Transfer the mixture to a spouted measuring cup or squeeze bottles. (Alternatively, use a liquid dropper or pipette to dispense.) Fill the molds to the top with the mixture and scrape excess fluid away.

4. Transfer the baking sheet with the molds to the refrigerator to chill for 2 hours, or until set. Release the gummies by pushing the candy outward from the back of the molds.

**STORAGE TIP:** Store in a resealable plastic bag in the refrigerator for up to 1 week.

**PREP TIP:** If little bear shapes aren't your thing, any silicone candy mold will work great. The red wine yields red gummies, while white wine and rosé gummies are colorless unless you add food dye. Pink food coloring mimics the rosy hue of rosé, but when using clear wine or spirits, consider using a color to match your party theme.

**PER SERVING (15 GUMMIES):** CALORIES: 49; TOTAL FAT: 0G; TOTAL CARBO-HYDRATES: 1G; FIBER: 0G; PROTEIN: 2G; SUGAR: 0G; SWEETENER CARBS: 14G

**MACROS:** FAT: 0%; PROTEIN: 66%; CARBS: 34%

# HARD LEMON MERINGUES

**MAKES 20 COOKIES | PREP TIME: 20 MINUTES / COOK TIME: 40 MINUTES, PLUS
1 TO 2 HOURS TO FIRM UP**

**GLUTEN-FREE, NUT-FREE, VEGETARIAN** ⸻

Sugar-free meringues are popular dessert fare in the keto world because of their low-carb count, accessible ingredients, and simple sweet flavors. A dollop of spiked lemon curd is added to each cookie to balance the sweetness. Keep your eye on the oven temperature when baking; low and slow is key to prevent cracking and excessive browning.

8 tablespoons (1 stick) unsalted butter

1¼ cups powdered erythritol, divided

½ cup freshly squeezed lemon juice

4 large eggs, separated, at room temperature

1 tablespoon vodka (optional)

¼ teaspoon cream of tartar

½ teaspoon vanilla extract

1. Preheat the oven to 250°F. Line two rimmed baking sheets with parchment paper or silicone baking mats.

2. In a small saucepan, melt the butter over low heat. Remove from the heat and whisk in ¾ cup of erythritol, the lemon juice, egg yolks, and vodka (if using). Place the pan over low heat and whisk for about 10 minutes, or until the mixture begins to thicken. Remove from the heat and cool to room temperature.

3. In a large bowl, with an electric mixer, beat the egg whites and cream of tartar on low for about 2 minutes, until frothy. Add the vanilla and continue beating. Add the remaining ½ cup of erythritol gradually, increase the mixer speed to high, and beat for 7 to 8 minutes, until stiff peaks begin to form.

4. Fill a piping bag with the meringue mixture. (Alternatively, use a resealable plastic bag with a small hole cut in the corner.) Pipe out 20 large round meringues. Scoop 1 tablespoon of the lemon curd onto the center of each meringue.

5. Bake for 20 minutes. Reduce the oven temperature to 200°F and bake for an additional 20 minutes. Turn the oven off and leave the meringues to rest in the oven for 1 to 2 hours, until they are firm and easily release from the parchment or silicone. Allow to cool before serving.

**PER SERVING (1 COOKIE):** CALORIES: 57; TOTAL FAT: 6G; TOTAL CARBOHYDRATES: 1G; FIBER: 0G; PROTEIN: 1G; SUGAR: 0G; SWEETENER CARBS: 12G

**MACROS:** FAT: 88%; PROTEIN: 6%; CARBS: 6%

**STORAGE TIP:** Store in an airtight container in a cool, dry place for up to 2 weeks.

# DARK CHOCOLATE COCONUT RUM TRUFFLES

**MAKES 24 TRUFFLES | PREP TIME: 20 MINUTES, PLUS AT LEAST 1 HOUR TO CHILL / COOK TIME: 10 MINUTES**

**GLUTEN-FREE, NUT-FREE, VEGETARIAN**

The chocolate ganache used to roll truffles can be a little finicky if it's too soft, so give it plenty of time to chill, and return the mixture to the refrigerator if the balls don't easily hold their shape. Coconut flavors are only one of many ways to enjoy this popular dessert; consider rolling the truffles in minced nuts or unsweetened cocoa powder for variety.

1 cup sugar-free dark chocolate baking chips

¼ cup coconut oil, unsalted butter, or ghee

¾ cup heavy cream

¼ cup powdered allulose or sweetener of choice

2 tablespoons rum

¼ teaspoon vanilla extract

¼ cup unsweetened shredded coconut

1. Fill a medium saucepan halfway with water and bring to a simmer over medium-low heat. Place the baking chips in a large heatproof bowl and set it over the simmering pot. Using a heat-resistant spatula, stir the chocolate until melted. Mix in the coconut oil.

2. In another medium saucepan, combine the cream, allulose, rum, and vanilla over medium heat until steaming. (Alternatively, heat the mixture in the microwave in a microwave-safe dish.)

3. Remove the bowl of chocolate mixture and the pan of cream mixture from the heat. Carefully pour the cream mixture into the bowl of chocolate mixture. Stir to combine well.

4. Transfer to a shallow pan for chilling and chill in the refrigerator for a minimum of 1 hour, or until the truffles are thick enough to hold their shape.

5. Line a rimmed baking sheet with aluminum foil. Shape tablespoon portions of the mixture into balls and roll in the shredded coconut to coat. Place on the baking sheet. Chill in the refrigerator to set the chocolate, but serve at room temperature.

STORAGE TIP: Store in an airtight container in the refrigerator for up to 2 weeks.

**PER SERVING (2 TRUFFLES):** CALORIES: 155; TOTAL FAT: 15G; TOTAL CARBOHYDRATES: 3G; FIBER: 2G; PROTEIN: 2G; SUGAR: 1G; SWEETENER CARBS: 4G

**MACROS:** FAT: 88%; PROTEIN: 4%; CARBS: 8%

# BOOZY POPS

**MAKES 6 ICE POPS | PREP TIME: 10 MINUTES, PLUS 6 HOURS TO FREEZE**

**DAIRY-FREE, GLUTEN-FREE, NUT-FREE, VEGAN** ————————————

This boozy frozen treat captures the famous rum, coconut, and lime flavor combination. But a case can be made for freezing any one of your favorite mixed drinks in an ice pop mold. Get creative with your hot-weather drinks and transform them into ice pops instead!

1 avocado, halved and pitted

1½ cups canned full-fat coconut milk, stirred

¼ cup crystallized allulose or sweetener of choice

2 ounces rum

1 ounce freshly squeezed lime juice

1. Scoop the avocado into a blender. Add the coconut milk, allulose, rum, and lime juice and process until smooth.

2. Fill 6 (4-ounce) ice pop molds with the mixture. Softly tap the molds on the counter to release air bubbles. Insert sticks in the center of each, then freeze for 6 hours, or until completely solid.

3. Store the frozen pops in the molds until ready to serve.

> **PREP TIP:** To serve, release each ice pop by rinsing the outside of the mold briefly under warm water.

**PER SERVING (1 ICE POP):** CALORIES: 195; TOTAL FAT: 17G; TOTAL CARBO-HYDRATES: 6G; FIBER: 3G; PROTEIN: 2G; SUGAR: 1G; SWEETENER CARBS: 8G

**MACROS:** FAT: 83%; PROTEIN: 5%; CARBS: 12%

# IRISH CREAM MOUSSE

**MAKES 4 DRINKS | PREP TIME: 10 MINUTES, PLUS 1 HOUR TO SET /
COOK TIME: 5 MINUTES**

**GLUTEN-FREE, NUT-FREE, VEGETARIAN**

With its rich, creamy flavors and surprisingly light and airy texture, this Irish cream mousse will feel self-indulgent. But without all of the extra sugar, you can enjoy the creamy liqueur flavors guilt-free in this dessert—a great way to satisfy your sweet tooth and catch a buzz.

¼ cup water

¼ cup crystallized allulose or sweetener of choice

2 tablespoons coconut oil, unsalted butter, or ghee

1 teaspoon instant coffee powder

1 teaspoon vanilla extract

1 teaspoon unsweetened cocoa powder

¼ cup Irish whiskey

1 cup heavy cream

1. In a large saucepan, combine the water, allulose, coconut oil, instant coffee, vanilla, and cocoa powder over medium heat until the sweetener has dissolved. Remove from the heat, stir in the whiskey, and allow the mixture to cool.

2. In a large bowl, with an electric mixer, whip the cream on medium for 7 to 8 minutes, until stiff peaks form. Fold in the cooled whiskey mixture.

3. Transfer to serving glasses or dessert dishes. Chill in the refrigerator to set for a minimum of 1 hour, or until ready to serve.

**PER SERVING:** CALORIES: 301; TOTAL FAT: 29G; TOTAL CARBOHYDRATES: 2G; FIBER: 0G; PROTEIN: 1G; SUGAR: 2G; SWEETENER CARBS: 12G

**MACROS:** FAT: 95%; PROTEIN: 2%; CARBS: 3%

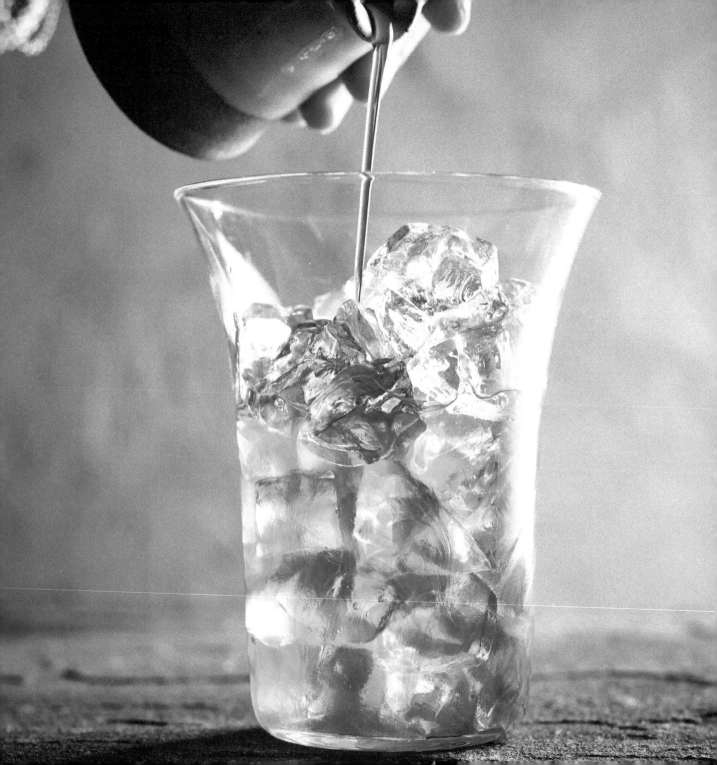

# MEASUREMENT CONVERSIONS

## VOLUME EQUIVALENTS (LIQUID)

| US STANDARD | US STANDARD | METRIC (APPROX.) |
|---|---|---|
| 2 tablespoons | 1 fl. oz. | 30 mL |
| ¼ cup | 2 fl. oz. | 60 mL |
| ½ cup | 4 fl. oz. | 120 mL |
| 1 cup | 8 fl. oz. | 240 mL |
| 1½ cups | 12 fl. oz. | 355 mL |
| 2 cups or 1 pint | 16 fl. oz. | 475 mL |
| 4 cups or 1 quart | 32 fl. oz. | 1 L |
| 1 gallon | 128 fl. oz. | 4 L |

## OVEN TEMPERATURES

| FAHRENHEIT (F) | CELSIUS (C) (APPROX.) |
|---|---|
| 250° | 120° |
| 300° | 150° |
| 325° | 165° |
| 350° | 180° |
| 375° | 190° |
| 400° | 200° |
| 425° | 220° |
| 450° | 230° |

## VOLUME EQUIVALENTS (DRY)

| US STANDARD | METRIC (APPROX.) |
|---|---|
| ⅛ teaspoon | 0.5 mL |
| ¼ teaspoon | 1 mL |
| ½ teaspoon | 2 mL |
| ¾ teaspoon | 4 mL |
| 1 teaspoon | 5 mL |
| 1 tablespoon | 15 mL |
| ¼ cup | 59 mL |
| ⅓ cup | 79 mL |
| ½ cup | 118 mL |
| ⅔ cup | 156 mL |
| ¾ cup | 177 mL |
| 1 cup | 235 mL |
| 2 cups or 1 pint | 475 mL |
| 3 cups | 700 mL |
| 4 cups or 1 quart | 1 L |

## WEIGHT EQUIVALENTS

| US STANDARD | METRIC (APPROX.) |
|---|---|
| ½ ounce | 15 g |
| 1 ounce | 30 g |
| 2 ounces | 60 g |
| 4 ounces | 115 g |
| 8 ounces | 225 g |
| 12 ounces | 340 g |
| 16 ounces or 1 pound | 455 g |

# RESOURCES

## WEBSITE

Ketogasm.com: Free keto recipes, meal plans, and resources. Visit Ketogasm.com/cocktails to join the newsletter.

## BOOK

*Keto: A Woman's Guide & Cookbook* by Tasha Metcalf: Learn more about the science behind ketogenic diets, hormonal balance, and weight loss for women.

# RECOMMENDED BRANDS

## SWEETENERS

Wholesome Yum Besti: allulose (crystallized and powdered), monk fruit (crystallized and powdered blend with allulose; granulated and powdered blend with erythritol), and erythritol (granulated and powdered)

## SPARKLING WATERS

Sparkling Ice Sparkling Water: intense fruit-flavored mixers, perfect as juice substitutes

Bubly Sparkling Water: for more subtle fruit flavors

## WATER FLAVORINGS

MiO

Stur

## ELECTROLYTE SUPPLEMENT

Elemental Labs LMNT Hydration Powder: to replenish electrolytes for hangover prevention

# REFERENCES

Brewery Ommegang. "Meet Ommegang Brut IPA, a Different Breed of Bubbly." Accessed April 29, 2020. ommegang.com/2018/11 /meet-ommegang-brut-ip a-a-different-breed-of-bubbly

Bridge Brewing Company. "Prime Time: No Compromises." Accessed April 29, 2020. bridgebrewing.com/prime-time

Brite Idea Foods, LLC. "H2wOw Flavors." Accessed April 29, 2020. h2wow.com

Comité Champagne. "Dosage, or 'liqueur d'expédition.'" Accessed April 16, 2020. www.champagne.fr /en/from-vine-to-wine/ wine-making/dosage

Devil's Backbone Brewing Company. "Bright Tangerine Sparkling Ale." Accessed April 29, 2020. dbbrewing company.com/beverage /bright-tangerine-sparkling-ale

Dogfish Head Craft Brewery Inc. "Slightly Mighty." Accessed April 29, 2020. dogfish.com/brewery/beer /slightly-mighty#fishgate-dialog

FitClick. "Grenache Red Wine-5 Fl Oz Svg." Accessed April 29, 2020. fitclick. com/how_many_calories_in_Grenache _Red_Wine_5_fl_oz_svg?fd=179674#. XvZKLpNKiyt

Hard Seltzer Beverage Company, LLC. "Find Your Favorite Truly." Accessed 29, 2020. trulyhardseltzer.com/flavors

Payne, Natasha E., J. Helen Cross, Josemir W. Sander, and Sanjay M. Sisodiya. "The ketogenic and related diets in adolescents and adults: a review." *Epilepsia* 52, no. 11 (2011): 1941–1948. doi:10.1111/j.1528-1167.2011.03287.x

United States Department of Agriculture. "FoodData Central." Accessed

April 29, 2020. fdc.nal.usda.gov
/index.html

Westman, Eric C., Richard D. Feinman,
John C. Mavropoulos, Mary C. Vernon,
Jeff S. Volek, James A. Wortman,
William S. Yancy, and Stephen D.
Phinney. "Low-carbohydrate nutrition
and metabolism." *American Journal
of Clinical Nutrition* 86, no. 2 (2007):

276–284. doi.org/10.1093
/ajcn/86.2.276

White Claw Seltzer Works. "Home."
Accessed April 29, 2020. whiteclaw
.com/#home

Wild Basin. "Wild Basin Boozy Sparkling Water." Accessed April 29, 2020.
wildbasinboozywater.com/#2

# INDEX

# ACKNOWLEDGMENTS

I have to start by thanking my drinking buddies—you know who you are. Who would have thought all those wild nights would come in handy for writing a book? Thanks for all the laughs, silly memories, and inside jokes.

Shout out to my partner, Bradley, for being a walking encyclopedia of bartending trivia and know-how. Thanks for letting me pick your brain and being such an eager recipe tester.

Mom, Dad, Tiff, Trev—thanks for cheering me on through these strange times. I love you guys!

And last, but certainly not least, I would like to thank my publisher and the hardworking team at Callisto Media for bringing this book together. To my editor, Anna Pulley, you are a total rockstar. Thank you for making my words shine; drinks are on me! Big hugs and high fives to everyone involved in getting this book out there. I'm honored to be part of the family. Let's do it again!

# ABOUT THE AUTHOR

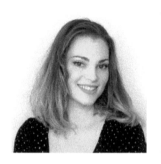

**Tasha Metcalf** is a writer, nutritionist, recipe developer, and founder of the wildly popular website Ketogasm.com. She creates healthy, down-to-earth recipes for low-carb and keto dietary patterns using accessible ingredients and unfussy techniques. Tasha also teaches the well-known Hello Keto course and online nutrition workshops. She lives in Tacoma, Washington, with her partner, Bradley, and their two amazing kiddos.

CPSIA information can be obtained
at www.ICGtesting.com
Printed in the USA
LVHW011117240121
677287LV00004B/4